The Anxious Mom Manifesto

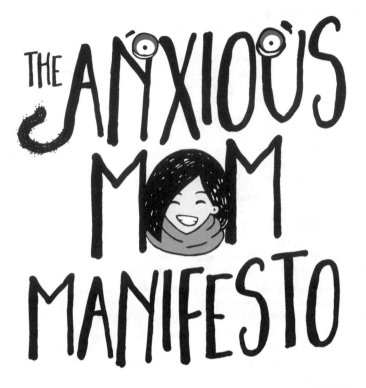

THE ANXIOUS MOM MANIFESTO

18 Lessons to Control Your Anxiety Monster

Paola B. Sur

Illustrations by Tatiana Williams

NEW YORK

LONDON • NASHVILLE • MELBOURNE • VANCOUVER

The Anxious Mom Manifesto

18 Lessons to Control Your Anxiety Monster

Published in New York, New York, by Morgan James Publishing. Morgan James is a trademark of Morgan James, LLC. www.MorganJamesPublishing.com

The Anxious Mom Manifesto is a book by Paola B. Sur, Chief Content Officer of **Momxious**, a platform created to offer encouragement, motivation, support and guidance through content and products for moms with anxiety.

All content and media on the **Momxious** Platform including this book is created and published for informational purposes only. **It is not intended to be a substitute for professional medical advice and should not be relied on as health or personal advice.**

Always seek the guidance of your doctor or other qualified health professional with any questions you may have regarding your health or a medical condition. Never disregard the advice of a medical professional, or delay in seeking it because of something you have read on this book.

If you think you may have a medical emergency, call your doctor, go to the nearest hospital emergency department, or call the emergency services immediately. If you choose to rely on any information provided by **Momxious**, you do so solely at your own risk.

External (outbound) links to other websites or educational material (e.g. pdf's etc…) that are not explicitly created by **Momxious** are followed at your own risk. Under no circumstances is **Momxious** responsible for the claims of third party websites or educational providers.

If you wish to seek clarification on the above matters please don't hesitate to get in touch with **Momxious** support@momxious.com

ISBN 9781631952487 paperback
ISBN 9781631952494 eBook
Library of Congress Control Number: 2020939813

Cover Concept by:
Corrina Roberts
Claudia Monroy

Cover & Interior Design by:
Chris Treccani
www.3dogcreative.net

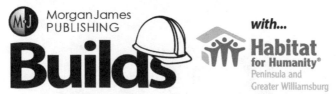

Morgan James is a proud partner of Habitat for Humanity Peninsula and Greater Williamsburg. Partners in building since 2006.

Get involved today! Visit
MorganJamesPublishing.com/giving-back

To all the moms that have touched my life, the mom friends who have been by my side in this wonderful journey, the moms that have shared their experiences and knowledge with me, my sisters in the fascinating world of motherhood.

Particularly I dedicate this book to the most wonderful mom in the world: mine.

Mami, este libro te lo dedico con todo mi amor. Gracias por tu esfuerzo y tus enseñanzas. Eres la luz que me ha guiado en esta tierra.

TABLE OF CONTENTS

SPECIAL ACKNOWLEDGMENTS

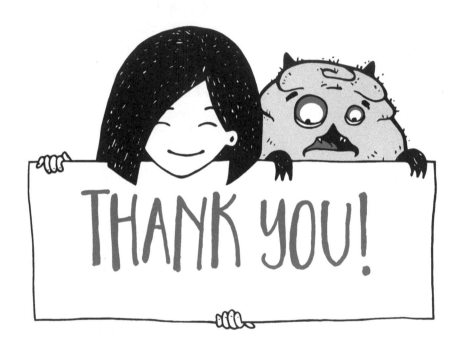

x | THE ANXIOUS MOM MANIFESTO

Thank you, God and my spirit guides who brought me to this very unique moment in my life, and allowed me to transmit these messages with love.

To my husband Igor Sur and my wonderful kids Eva and Erik. Your love is my light. Thank you for encouraging and understanding me always. My heart is forever yours and your love motivates me day by day.

To my supportive family and those amazing friends that are always cheering me up. Thank you for being there for me.

To Irina Sur, this project wouldn't have been possible without you. I am eternally grateful for your support and love.

To Michael Ebeling and Tabitha Moore. Thank you for helping me become aware of the endless possibilities of my future writing career.

To Keyla Medina-Rosa for the input and care while editing this book. I am so happy we got to work together again.

To Carolina Rico for appearing in my life in the right moment, guiding me to discover my purpose.

To Tatiana Williams and Claudia Monroy, my partners in crime:

Tatiana, you have been there from day 0 and I can't express my gratitude for being by my side all of these years, and for being my Victor Frankenstein to my Mary Shelly! Thanks to you "It's alive! It's alive!"

Claudia, your brilliance is beyond comprehension, to the point I think you might not even be human but like those extraterrestrial beings camouflaged among us in *Men in Black*! I have learned so much from you and nothing of what Momxious has accomplished so far could have been possible without you. This is just the beginning.

To Corrina Roberts for your extraordinary talent and fresh visual ideas that you are bringing into Momxious. Also for that beautiful cover design.

To Andres Rodriguez and Andres Cadavid for your contributions and help to our team.

And last but not least,

To David Hancock, Jim Howard, Bonnie Rauch, and the entire team at **Morgan James Publishing** for welcoming me to your family. It took me years to receive that call that is every author's dream come true. And I am so happy it came from you.

PREFACE

First Things First: Why I Gave My Anxiety Monster a Name and Why You Should Do It Too

Some people deal with skeletons in the closet. Ghosts haunt others. But for us, the ones suffering from anxiety, we need to battle with monsters; this is what anxiety is, a beast that you try to defeat every day, but instead, you might end up feeding it, nurturing it, and making it stronger and scarier.

I have my anxiety monster. For a while, I was trying not even to acknowledge its presence. I didn't understand what kind of monster it was; I just knew it appeared out of nowhere, and its unpredictable behavior was making me fear it more a more. I didn't know how to defeat it, and I guess I didn't even want to try. Until the day I named it. Triggerion I called it because I discovered it only appeared when something in me triggered it. I have been trying to make the monster disappear for years, unsuccessfully. Until after many attempts, I realized maybe it was not going anywhere. I had to come to terms with the idea that it might be around for a while or forever. This assertion was a challenging thing to accept. Anxiety can bring much uncertainty into your life when all you want to feel is a sense of security. One thing I was sure about, I was too tired of leaving in fear of its presence. The more you fear the monster, the bigger it gets. It all starts with that choice when you decide fear is no longer the path you want to follow.

In my search for certainty, I look for something I was comfortable with. I have been a dreamer and a writer for as long as I can remember. I turned to my creativity and abilities as a fantasy writer, to allow my mind to wander and look for inspirations and solutions to cope with fear. It hit me, like a strike of thunder. What if the monster was something I could see, what if I give it the traits of a character in my life to be able to understand my relationship with it? I wanted to use the personification mechanism cathartically. I was trying to think of it as something out of a cartoon rather than from a horror movie. Somehow, I needed it to be relatable and not particularly scary. By transforming it into something external to me and giving it specific traits, I realized that I could also own it. After all, I was the one giving it the powers necessary to control me, and it was winning. But I was ready to become the heroine of my story and not the victim, so I decided to imagine myself also like one of those heroic characters I depict in my epic novels. The hero that tamed the monster became my new motif. I was ready to release the fear and become the heroine I was always dreaming of being. My new relationship with Triggerion, which took me through a path of open and fresh wounds, showed me how to heal and reinvent myself, which has awoken the warrior powers inside me and made me write this book for others to see how this is possible.

Writing this book was not the only time I have used my love for the fantasy genre to find ways to cope with situations. Through all my life, I have turned to fantasy books for more than an escape mechanism. I believe fantasy stories can give us great perspectives of the world we live in. Through this book, you will also find inspirational quotes from beloved and famous fantasy characters. Additionally, you will see references to some of my favorite fantasy and science fiction stories and even a few pop culture associations. Ever since I created Triggerion, my life has changed in ways I can't possibly describe. During this transformation process, I also gave birth to a new fantasy book, *An Incredible World*, previously to writing *The Anxious Mom Manifesto*. I am assuming that the book also entails a great deal of my recovery process through its characters. But it's a trilogy that I haven't finished yet, so if you are interested in that, stay tuned.

The past couple of years before deciding on writing this book, I spent months on a deep soul searching, using Triggerion, among other things. While finding answers, I had to relive my whole journey in this battle, coming to the painful realization that I had suffered from anxiety all my life. However, I was unaware of that. Truth is my monster has been following me since childhood, but I didn't get the diagnose until my late 20s. The lack of knowledge of what I was suffering from probably made things worse, that's why I now have an intense commitment to creating awareness, and this book is part of that. I also recognized that anxiety was not always present. At some stages in my life, the monster would disappear for a while only to come back in full force. I needed to understand that, and how I was allowing that to happen. For sure, getting the diagnosis represented a significant change in my life. It was in 2006, or as I call it "The Year When Hell Broke Loose." Back then, I thought I was at the peak of my journalistic career; I felt that nothing could stop me. I was in a great relationship, and my friends were working with me on a personal project, so what could go wrong? Well... things started to fall like a house of cards.

I won't get into many details, but the project suddenly failed, and from there, the rest of the things started to fall apart. I was a complete mess, made many mistakes, and of course, my anxiety got extremely high. Then, Triggerion appeared after years of being dormant bringing all my insecurities, dizziness spells, insomnia, irrational fears, everything that I had experienced since childhood, and I couldn't understand. I was far away from my family, trying to build back my life. Until finally, a doctor explained it to me: "You have Generalized Anxiety Disorder (GAD)." After the diagnosis, everything changed. I think now those words could have had a significant impact on my life if I heard them earlier on, but I am a believer that everything has a reason when the time is right. So, after knowing that I had a condition I understood it could be treatable and effectively manageable. I didn't know how difficult it would be to do it.

I have tried different treatments, methods, foods, meditation, medication, therapy, reading books, articles, journals, and yes, I can say the monster was at bay sometimes, but it never truly disappeared. However, thanks to all of those things I tried I got a lot of tools on how to deal with it, and make it more controllable. The monster was the unwelcome guest in my life. I could be taking a shower, driving, working out, or even sleeping. Suddenly it was coming out of nowhere, disrupting my life. Sometimes it was easy to deal with it. Others I ended up in the ER... But something happened that changed things completely for me, something that gave me a spin, unlike any other event in my life: Motherhood.

Becoming a mother changes everything, including this. For the past nine years, my anxiety became a family issue affecting not only me but also those I love the most. I survived the first years of motherhood anxiety free. Or so I thought. In reality, anxiety was always there lurking like the shark on *Jaws* (cue the music!) Suddenly I was there again with panic attacks and the whole anxiety shenanigans. Then came that day I decided it was enough. The monster had taken a lot from me, and I was not going to allow it to take away the possibility to enjoy my children and my life as an adult. Among a lot of things, I started to write about it to cope. I created a blog series called *Momxious* and it was then when I decided to name the monster creating a character that embodied all that I was feeling. It not only has helped me immeasurably but also, has inspired me creatively. Through the beast, I have been able to analyze my experiences with anxiety differently. In this book, I will explain how I have done it and how other moms can do the same. I will give you my monster, my lessons, and my tools so you can also name it however you want and work your anxiety through it in a similar way as I did.

Here I will reveal some painful experiences as well as funny personal episodes; I will share what I have learned down the road and let you know how naming the monster helped me. Ultimately, this book came to life thanks to my realization that I didn't want my monster to get in my way of being the fulfilled mom I wanted to be. Please don't take me wrong. You can be an excellent mom and suffer from anxiety. It happens because life happens, but I knew I needed to find a solution, a more permanent solution so that I could be more present in my children's life.

As you read my journey, you will understand it has been more of a transformation, acknowledging the monster is there, but not giving it more power to control me while I stop fearing its presence. I realized I had to face it, and it was going to be a lonely battle. Even though I sometimes need somebody to talk to when I have these episodes, in the end, I am my only superhero. Nobody is going to rescue me. I can have sidekicks, you know, a Robin, a Chewbacca, or I can have my prince charming kissing me at the end of the day, but none of them are going to defeat Triggerion for me. Yes, my family gives me the most motivation to recover. But I know they can't make my monster disappear.

Now, this is very important before you embark on this journey with me. I am not writing this book to tell you a miracle cure for anxiety. I want to encourage you, motivate you, and inspire you. But I am not a psychologist, a therapist, or a doctor. I strongly advise you that if you are suffering from anxiety or any other mental health symptoms, talk to your doctor about it. Also you will find additional resources on my website momxious.com and social media accounts that might help you. If you are having thoughts of suicide or self-harm, call 911 or go to the nearest emergency room right away. You can also call the National Suicide Prevention Lifeline at 1-800-273-8255 to talk and find support 24/7.

What I offer here is my story: think of me as part of your mom tribe, a friend that is talking to you on a more personal level. Maybe my story is relatable to you and can help you in different ways. With this book, I intend to let you know that even when you have to fight your monster by yourself, at the same time, you are not alone. There are millions of us fighting the same battle in this exact moment. Maybe some of my words resonate with you, or you'd like to try some of my methods and exercises. I invite you to join me and hear what I have to say, and maybe you can also turn your monster into a master as I did. Anxiety can make you stronger, and I am proof of that.

Another goal is to contribute to the conversation about mental health. If you are reading this, you understand what I am saying. Having a mental condition shouldn't be taboo. Motherhood is too hard, and you know how judgmental our circles are (unfortunately.) We need to break that wheel by talking about this!!! (now I sound like Daenerys Targaryen) We shouldn't be afraid, and moms should help each other in any way we can, even if we only have words to offer.

I want to end this introduction giving props to Tatiana Williams, one of my best friends, and excellent mom and illustrator that perfectly captured how I felt and transformed my vision, my monster, into a visual reality. Thanks to her creativity and that special connection we share, Triggerion now has a face; and this helped me tremendously. Also my gratitude to Claudia Monroy, another great friend, and talented designer who has helped me to turn *Momxious* into a visual world of messages and a platform that is growing. Both of you are a fundamental part of this and I have no words to express my gratitude for all that you have done.

Now go ahead I give you permission to take its image, give it your own name. Color it differently if you want to! Now it is also yours.

Last but not least, I have to tell you about the manifesto. Writing the 18 rules or declarations was an easy task, but it had taken me years to figure each of those points out. I understand now how different my life would have been if I had known about this condition earlier. However, each one of us has unique life experiences, and that has a purpose. So at this moment, I am grateful that everything happened the way it did. Now all I want is to contribute to the conversation, so I want to talk about anxiety, share what I have learned, and ultimately support other moms that are in the same boat, so let's start sailing together.

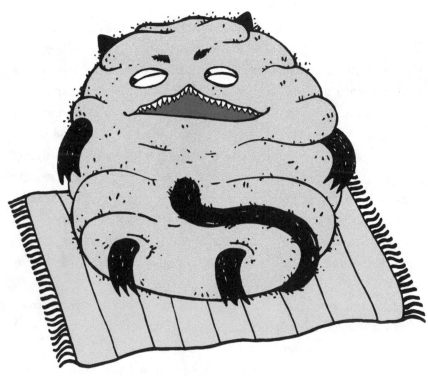

Name Your Monster

ANXIETY DOESN'T MAKE YOU A BAD MOM

 "A bruise is a lesson... and each lesson makes us better."
—**Arya Stark, Game of Thrones**

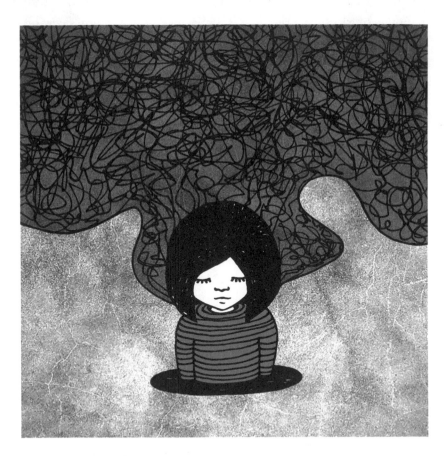

1

There is a question that people always ask me when I tell them I suffer from severe anxiety and panic attacks. "So, how does it feel?" I tell you one thing; **it is the most challenging thing to explain, and if you have never suffered from anxiety, it's complicated to understand.** Also, it's challenging because, for every person, the experience is different.

Let me try to explain for example, how a panic attack feels to me. It can happen at any moment. I could be driving or watching a movie or sleeping. Yes, it has happened when I am sleeping. Then out of the blue, I feel a hot flash, and then I start feeling dizzy. I immediately think that I am going to faint. That dull sensation starts a chain reaction in my brain, releasing a bunch of other stressful random thoughts that create a massive mess in my head. "What if it's something else, like a heart attack?" "What if I go back to sleep and I never wake up?" "What if I faint and I crash?" Then those thoughts get tangled. In seconds, all of the messages that I have created, all at the same time, all colliding with each other while I desperately try to find a resolution, sink me into a messy hole.

Then comes the guilt after the symptoms subside. I am always thinking, "But why? I have a good life. What is wrong with me?" All of this feels ten times worse when one of those episodes happens in front of my kids.

Once, some time ago, I was a mess. The panic attacks were frequently coming. I had to explain to my kids what was happening to me. Before I was a mother, if I had a panic attack or I was feeling anxious, I would seclude myself for a while. Now things were different. Panic attack or not, I still needed to be a parent, responsible for these two little human beings and their survival and security. I was so scared all the time, not only from the anxiety itself but also, thinking that I was passing the condition to them. I figured I could make the monster useful, so I used it to tell them about anxiety. I showed them its picture and explained to them that mommy sometimes felt sick. I reassured them that they should not be afraid when these situations happened because mommy could recover; mommy was not in danger. It was funny when Eva, my oldest one, mentioned that it looked cute, "He looks like from *Monsters Inc.*," she said. She made me realize with that comment that monsters not always have to scare us. We can see them and learn not to fear them. (Who knew? There is still wisdom in those animated movies.)

I also told them what to do when mommy was scared by the monster. Eva knows what to say to me and what to do. She starts telling me a story, or holds my hand if she can, and reminds me to breathe and drink water. Erik, my youngest, still has no full comprehension of the whole thing, but he knows that it will pass and he doesn't freak out. Another time, in one of those birthday party goodie bags that are useless most of the time, Erik got a stress ball with a soft pointy surface. I started using it all the time, particularly when I was getting anxious. Many times, when they saw me stressing out or knew I was getting anxious, they looked for it all over the house and gave it to me. I have come to replace that stress ball many times now. I also talked to their teachers about this situation, in case they see any reaction I should be aware of. So far, they are doing fine.

It was not always that easy, though. One of the most significant challenges of coping while being a mom was hiding my emotions from the kids. You never want them to be scared, or that they can misinterpret what it's happening to you. The thing is that anxiety can make you react in unexpected ways. The most usual for me was crying uncontrollably or yelling. It still happens and when it does sometimes is extremely difficult for me. Mainly because of the guilt that I feel afterward. Yelling at them happened frequently. One day my daughter told me she was scared of me, and it broke my heart to pieces. Controlling those emotions is hard. The good thing is that you can recognize it's your anxiety talking and not you. Don't be ashamed when this happens. There are no more understanding creatures than your kids. They see you with love, no matter what. Talking with them about your anxiety will make your relationship better, plus there is no better response than a hug from one of your kids. If you lose control, don't leave like that. Once you calm down, make sure they understand where your reaction came from so they won't feel guilty.

Slowly I started letting the guilt go away. Sometimes it comes with the monster, but I am not making this sensation to rule my life anymore. The truth is that motherhood and guilt are married. It's a fact. There is so much pressure that we put on ourselves every day — so many expectations. I realized the main problem is that we have trouble handling the ugliness of motherhood. Before you start throwing stones at me, please continue reading. Yes, motherhood has an ugly side; and it has nothing to do with what you feel for your family or you think about motherhood overall.

Moms get tired, burned, bored, sick, worried, depressed, and fed up. Because we are not angels, we are humans. Motherhood is incredibly overwhelming, no matter the kind of mom you are or the amount or lack of help you have. Moms need to wear different hats throughout the day, and sometimes we don't have the energy or patience to do all so lovingly. Some can cope with all of this without the anxiety disorder, and I envy them, and God knows I do. But for others like me, the ones that have to deal with the anxiety monster and panic attacks on top of it, that ugly side and guilt can create a dark repetitive cycle. There is something you need to repeat yourself every day: **It's ok not to be ok. You don't**

have to be the perfect mom, and your kids don't have to be the perfect kids. Perfection doesn't coexist with motherhood. Forget about it! Always look for progress and how can your reactions get better and better.

My fellow anxious mom, I understand you and let me say something: You are NOT crazy. You are NOT weak. Anxiety is exhausting and challenging, but you can overcome this. It's a process. It might take time, and that is fine. Don't be afraid to open up, to ask for help. I know that it is so difficult to explain this to people that have no clue what a panic attack is. Let alone explain this to your kids. But I can assure you, it is more common than you think and you will find those who will listen to you, give you a hand, a piece of advice, or love you and let you know they are there for you. I know you are trying to avoid embarrassment and judgment. But don't let those feelings get in the way of recovering your peace. Anxiety doesn't define you or dictate how good of a mother you are. We are all learning, trying our best. And the simple fact to acknowledge that you want to recover and get better from this makes you a great human, a great mom. I recognize the strength in you because I know it's not easy to overcome those episodes while protecting and raising your kids.

So from an anxious mom to another, I will tell you one more thing: We can do this! We have endured pregnancies, late-night feedings, diaper changing, awful playdates, toddler years to name a few, of course, we can kick the panic attacks and the anxiety monster in the butt too.

LESSON: Anxiety doesn't define you or what kind of mother you are. Don't let guilt consume your thoughts and give credit to yourself just for the fact that you are willing to recover.

 TIPS:

- Don't hide your anxiety from your loved ones. Find ways to explain to them in the best way you can about how you feel, and what to do, and most importantly, what do you expect from them. Don't be afraid to talk to your kids about this. They are smarter than you think and they can be incredibly understanding.
- Speak about the ugliness of motherhood. Yes, it is lovely how we post our perfect pictures and to brag about all the milestones online, but we need to tell other mothers about the dark side of the moon too. Let's not perpetuate the perfection standard of motherhood.
- If you need help, ask for help. Don't feel ashamed. All human beings deal with something different. Moms need help sometimes because we are not angels; we are humans.

YOU HAVE THE POWER TO GIVE THE TOXIC OR HEALING VALUE TO THOSE AROUND YOU

"We must all face the choice between what is right and what is easy."
— Albus Dumbledore, *Harry Potter and the Goblet of Fire*

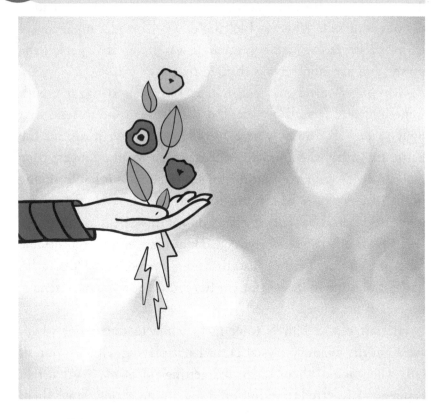

ince I was a child, I developed a fear of public speaking. I can say with 100% certainty that I had some panic attacks and anxiety episodes triggered by this specific scenario but I didn't know it then. It's still something I keep working on, and maybe that's why I chose writing as my primary means of communication with others. I am not sure what I fear about it. Most likely is related to a fear of being judged and it goes deeper than that. One day as I was trying to get out of a bad panic attack, triggered by an ugly comment that I received from a friend that kept bothering me for days, I suddenly became irrationally angry. Still, I was not mad at her but at myself. Why was I letting that person ruin my recovery with one single negative comment? I was giving that person the power, and my monster was thrilled that day.

My anger made me realize that I've been struggling with something stronger all my life and that it was time to send that fight to hell. Far away, where I could never find it again: The battle to justify who I am to others, which for the longest time marked my life and my relationships, and perhaps it has been one of the biggest causes of my anxiety. Early on, I developed a need to please others. I have always been one of those people concerned about what others would say or think of me and got comfortable following another person's lead instead of me being the leader. It's like not wanting to drive your car but rather let someone else take control of the wheel.

It started as a kid. It took me a while to remember when, but I got the memory crystal clear. I was playing with a group of girls when one of them suggested getting rid of me. "What had happened?" I started thinking I did something wrong. Since then, I was timid and was (still is) very difficult for me to make new friends. Because in the back in my mind, I was thinking "people at some point will want to get rid of me." I became timider and afraid to interact with others. I figured out it was more comfortable if I could do things or act in a way they expected so I could be accepted. By making that decision, I shouted down the possibility of exploring who I was. Instead, I chose to hide behind other people's shadows, creating a narrative about myself that I believed in for years and years to come. This is what happens sometimes; you make a set of beliefs about yourself, and you stick with them because it is easy, even if they are not true at all.

It continued happening as a teenager. I was struggling to identify myself and craved to be accepted; this is a battle that all of us have at a certain point in our lives. I always felt like an outsider. But when I imitated other's behaviors and followed their leads, I noticed nobody questioned me. At that time, I must say that despite having several friendships, few people knew me. All I was doing was playing a role without realizing it, all while secretly, I was putting labels on myself to make things easier. I began to create a narrative, a story about myself that others could accept. The shy, quiet girl that nobody could figure out. The faithful friend who went out of her way to see others happy but not herself. That was me.

What's more upsetting now is to think that girl thought she was ugly, graceless, and invisible, only because she found out that some boys in the class had made a list ranking the girls' beauty and finding out they put her on the very bottom. Kids can be cruel; we learn that very early. And now, as a mom, it terrifies me. I always tell my kids not to be afraid of showing who they are or be ashamed of what they like or dislike. In my case, for example, very few people knew things about me back then, like that I was a soccer fan, or that I liked fantasy literature and dreamed of writing stories similar to those I consumed, nor that I was a fervent fan of *Star Wars*. Yes, I was a nerd, and I tried my best to hide that for fear of being judged because back then, being a nerd was "not cool." I was like those kids on *Stranger Things*, and my *Demogorgon* was anxiety. It was easier to be the girl that no one pays attention to, although that hurt a little in solitude.

I left high school, wanting to get rid of that role. Nevertheless, I ended up putting even more labels on. I studied to become a journalist, and the story that I lived as a teenager I repeated it in college. I put on several masks, although I must admit that I found significant friendships in this time of my life, people with whom I could just be me. When I graduated more than 20 years ago, I imagined having a very different experience than the one I have now in my 40s. I left my country, Colombia, as soon as I graduated, tired of labels, and eager to seek my happiness elsewhere. I achieved a lot as a journalist. Despite how difficult it's to leave the country where you are born and grow up, in the United States, I found new friendships and a voice. I also met who would be my future husband, so you could say I was having a happy and fulfilled life. So why did I still felt that emptiness? Instead of accepting my authenticity, what I was doing was putting on conventional labels, and the more tags, the bigger the emptiness. It was no coincidence that my diagnosis let to an explosion of anxiety.

There is always a spark that ignites your fire and opens our eyes. I found comfort in something I had left forgotten in the corner of my soul. I sat down to write and that's how *The Lake of Miracles,* my first book, and novel, was born. The simple fact of finishing it made me realize that I never really wanted an executive career in media, something I was convinced it was my right path to follow. However, I always wanted to be a writer. But thousands of questions drowned that dream, and the bad thing is that they were not my questions but those of others. Many did it to my face; others let me see their judgment in their eyes. How could I leave a promising media career for a "simple hobby"? How could I make a living from writing, and how would I help my husband with household finances if writing books do not leave a penny?

Motherhood added to the spark. It gave me more strength to pursue my dreams and to accept who I really was, or at least it was there when I started to get rid of the labels and to embrace my authenticity. I managed to finish a Master's Degree and I finally managed to publish my book against all the odds. Meanwhile, the questions of others continued. "Where do you get the money to travel?" "What do you do all day at home?" "Why you don't get a stable job if your children already go to school?" and the list went on...

A few months ago I found some spiritual advice that made me realize that my mistake had been trying to please the rest of the planet and not myself all my life. The moment you remove the masks you have had on to please others and let your pure self flow, your life starts to change. It has been months of introspection and of recognizing that although my true self showed from time to time, I never let it come out, until the moment I decided enough was enough. It's never too late. No matter which life stage you are, embrace authenticity, and grab your dreams.

Amid my crying episode regarding the "ugly comment" that I described before, I understood all of this more clearly, of course when my anger subsided. We will never be able to silence the prejudices of others; we will always have to listen to their questions, the advice that we have never asked for, their requests and demands, their expectations of us. It's something that we cannot control. What we can do is learn to listen, receive the good, and when it hurts reject the bad. Just imagine yourself as a colander, others can be light in our lives or can intoxicate us. It depends on what we allow to get through inside us. We are human beings that need from each other to move forward. Some come into our lives and sporadically leave, others stay, others hurt you, others shine on you. For someone who suffers from anxiety, it is difficult to find that balance of managing what comes from others but isn't impossible.

We need to talk. Anxiety is not something that we have to swallow forever. Many people will judge when you decide to speak. However, there will always be someone willing to listen to you. And whoever loves you and does not understand what anxiety is, will at least make an effort. To those with someone who suffers from anxiety and do not know what I am talking about, I can only say that we never look for or need to be fixed. We do not need to hear that everything will be fine. We do not need your judgments; if you do not know anxiety, the best you can do to help someone you love is educating yourself about it. If there is something we need, it's love. A hug at the right moment can get us out of a state of panic. A call can distract us from chaos. A visit reminds us that we are not alone in this world. There is much we can learn from anxiety to be better human beings, compassionate, and full of light to give.

Be who you are. It's that simple, with anxiety and all. We are a beautiful mix of things with different colors and meanings. Accept who you are, and don't be afraid to explore it. You cannot control what others say or think, but you have the power in you to make those comments, questions, and judgments nurture or intoxicate you. Make a choice.

LESSON: We cannot control what others say or think. But we can control how it will affect us and react accordingly. Always accept who you are and let that person flourish.

TIPS:

- Remember: Be a colander. Let the light go through and throw the garbage away.
- Be as clear as possible. Tell others about the support you need in the event of an episode, so they will know what to say or do.
- Have an **Anxiety Distractor Buddy**. Choose a person you can talk to when you have a panic attack or have an anxiety episode, he or she can help you go through it with breathing exercises, or sending you funny GIFS or messages. Sometimes a good chat will help you when you need support. You can have several ADBs if you want and yes you can include your pet!
- Identify your energy vampires and try to avoid them or cut them from your life. You know who I am talking about, those people that are just merely toxic. Stay away from those.

NURTURE YOUR MIND, BODY AND SOUL

"All we have to decide is what to do with the time that is given us."
— **Gandalf, _Lord of the Rings_**

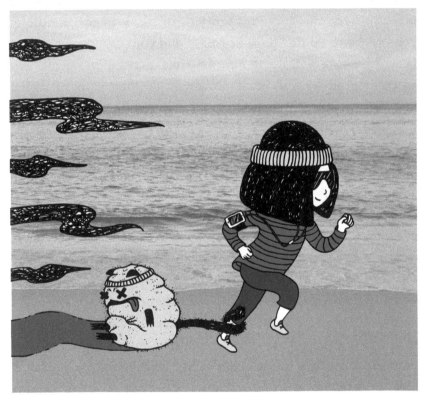

15

One of the first pieces of advice you receive when you mention your anxiety to others is to do exercise, which has some logic behind. When you exercise, your body releases endorphins, a chemical process that triggers positive feelings and overall is right for your body and mind. Sounds easy, right? Well, let me tell you. For some of us anxiety sufferers, even trying to do something you know will be good for your body, can be a struggle. Even while exercising, the mischievous monster can sneak in the middle of your workout, raining on your parade and your efforts of trying to be healthier. Also, motherhood sometimes gets in the way. It's not an excuse, but it's a reality, especially in the first years of raising our kids we struggle to find time for ourselves. In this chaotic scenario, we, the anxious moms, yearn for balance but this is the most challenging thing to find when you have thousands of tasks to do plus all the demands of life, adding mister monster laughing at us like *Pennywise* in the corner of the room.

I used to enjoy exercising without problems. After my first daughter was born, it took me less than a year to get back in shape, and soon I was feeling like myself again. The second time around, things were **completely** different. I gained much more weight, I had less time for myself, and I was exhausted **all** the time. If I have to confess, I think the first year of being a mom of two has been one of the hardest years of my life, something I will address in more detail in a future chapter. My inability to get in shape, plus my struggles with motherhood made me a person I didn't recognize, literally. I didn't like the person I saw in the mirror and I didn't like the person inside either. I was depressed and anxious; until one day I decided to start running; not entirely like *Forrest Gump* and not like running away from my problems. I just decided to give running as an activity a try.

Stop right there. Don't even think this is one of those stories you read in fitness magazines when the person tells you how running made them lose 150 pounds and then proceed to show you the pictures of before and after. I am not even close to my pre-Erik shape and weight and he is seven years old. Running has not taken me there yet; however, it turned out to be a great tool to fight my anxiety monster.

I started running 5ks. I remember that after I finished my first one, I felt like I just had come back from war. But with time, I started learning how to train, and I now enjoy running on the beach and try longer races from time to time. Also, I have to say runners high is something that is entirely accurate!

Recently I joined a running club, and let me tell you something: The running community is one of the most encouraging groups you can ever find. I am not the fastest, and the only rule in my journey to become a better person is not allowing myself to compete with other people but myself. Beating my records, running a little bit faster, becoming stronger, those are my goals. I don't care what other people do in the gym or post on social media. What I love about running is, however, that at that time I can connect with my inner-self. As my physical body gets tired, my mind starts to get brighter. I am not sure how but plenty of my inspiration has come after a run. At that moment, I have conversations with myself. I listen to the music I like and let my mind wander. I forget that there is a world spinning around and people passing by. I am in my world, and nobody can get in to disrupt it.

I still have a battle with my body image, and it has been tough for me to get back in shape, or at least in a way that I am entirely comfortable. For the past years, my weight has had a yo-yo effect, in part thanks to anxiety, because there are periods that I simply just don't want to exercise at all. Plus, sometimes I can't keep away from the refrigerator. I work from home, and there are days that my anxiety makes me open the fridge like every hour. The monster wins some battles; it happens. What I try to do is aiming for progress, not perfection. I stopped weighing myself. It was messing with my head a lot. I use my intuition (and my clothes) as a gage. With time, I started to be more comfortable with the way I look, and I keep trying to be healthier. I forgive myself for those moments when I can't and move on.

Another issue I was having was getting panic attacks in the middle of workouts. But I feel great satisfaction when I decide to drag my anxiety monster along and show it that I can do this even when it decides to show up. Every time I finish a race, or even a complete Zumba or spinning class, I feel I am moving forward, and I am getting better.

Some weeks are better than others, and some workouts are better than others. But when I have those anxiety episodes that drain me physically and mentally, I give myself a couple of days to relax and do nothing. Then I come back, and I kick my anxiety monster's butt. I think the key is finding an activity that you enjoy. Don't do it because of others but because it feels right for you. You may have to try a few things before you find the workout that makes you happy. Don't give up on trying.

However, there's more than just taking care of your body. You need to find ways for your mind and your soul to join the party too. There's too much negativity in the world; all you have to do is turn on the news. And let's not even begin with the social media conversation. I won't tell you to get disconnected from the world. You can't live in a bubble, especially because you need information on what's going on in the world to be a guide for your kids. What you can do is find a balance on what you consume daily. You know that you have to nurture your body with healthy foods and exercise. So does your mind and soul. You need to find ways to keep them stimulated, alive, and nurtured.

What I try to do is surround myself with books about topics and genres I care passionately. Sometimes the audiobooks work wonders, while you do house chores or when you are driving to pick up the kids, or any "free time" and by free, I mean you are not nurturing or attending your little humans, you need to try to spend it in nurturing you. Entertainment is also crucial. Your mind needs an escape. That is the reason why I think there is more than marketing brilliance on the "Netflix and chill" phrase, be it a getaway with family, a trip with friends, lunch with a coworker, drinks with the girls... Entertainment is vital for your mind but is even more critical not to feel guilty when you spend time like this. As I said, it is all about balance, and this doesn't mean you are unattending your family. On the contrary, if you are happy and relaxed, everyone will benefit.

Your soul is a little more complicated because that is a VERY PERSONAL road. Only you can identify how to keep your soul balanced, but for some meditation is the path. Yes, yes, I know. An anxious person meditating? Are you kidding? I used to have tremendous resistance to it. But so I did with running, and now I can't live without either-or. When I finally decided to give meditation a try, I realized tons of guides and apps promise you the perfect meditation practice. The truth is you have to try and try and try until you find something that resonates with you. Remember those times when your baby didn't seem to calm down, and you tried everything out there no matter how ridiculous the idea might have sound, to find out it was the sound of the laundry dryer that made him fall asleep (true story)? If that example doesn't work for you, think about meditation like a type of diet. Some people use Keto; some people like The South Beach Diet; this is how I feel meditation works. Some practices speak to you, and others simply don't. There is mindfulness meditation, Kundalini mantras, and others have great results with swearing meditation! So, keep trying because when you find the one that works for you, the experience can be amazing. You can even mix them up. Whatever works for you.

Anxiety can efficiently disconnect you from your soul because many times, you feel like you are dark inside. There is no light in you to give. No energy. And it is in these moments when your monster feasts. It loves when you are disconnected because it gets the power to control your emotions. These are the moments in which it tells you lies, such as you are not worthy, you can't do this, you don't deserve love, you are weak, you are alone, and you believe all of it. Make sure when one of these lies appears, you can identify that your monster is speaking, and trying to keep you disconnected.

More than the body or the mind, I think finding that balance within your soul is the most challenging part but also the most important. However, don't give up searching. If praying helps you, pray. If believing in something helps you, feel it. I don't want to lecture you on this one. As I said, this is very personal. For example, I come from a Catholic family, so of course, my first impulse is to pray. In my search for finding a balance with my soul, I started reading about energies, angels, and spirit guides, and it has helped me tremendously. Sometimes praying the Rosary is a meditation for me or even listening to it (yes, there is an app for this.) I am not asking you to follow my beliefs; It's your decision and your path. I am just telling you my experience. I knew something was missing, and I know you feel it too, so I started searching until I found the philosophies and practices that nurture my soul. You can do this too.

Now I know that everything you do toward finding your balance, nurturing your body, mind, and soul signifies progress. It doesn't have to be 24/7. You need to indulge sometimes as well, and of course, you can't follow a perfect nurturing mind, body, and soul practice all the time. But small things here and there make the difference. Soon you will start cultivating healthier habits without effort. And progress makes you feel better one day at a time.

LESSON: Nurture your body, mind, and soul to find a balance following your path. But remember this is a personal endeavor and you are the only one who can unveil it.

TIPS:

- Find activities that you like and that won't feel forced on you. Remember it has to be fun.
- Don't be afraid to explore things and try new methods. Resistance can be the monster telling you lies.
- If you have to compete, compete with yourself.
- Balance is also a reconnection with your passions. So, explore your passions.
- Take it one day at a time.
- If you feel overwhelmed or exhausted physically, mentally, or emotionally, give yourself a break. Do something different for a couple of days, or do nothing at all! You'll come back to it.

USE THE RESOURCES THAT WORK BETTER FOR YOU

"Just keep swimming. Just keep swimming. Just keep swimming, swimming, swimming. What do we do? We swim, swim."

—Dory, *Finding Nemo*

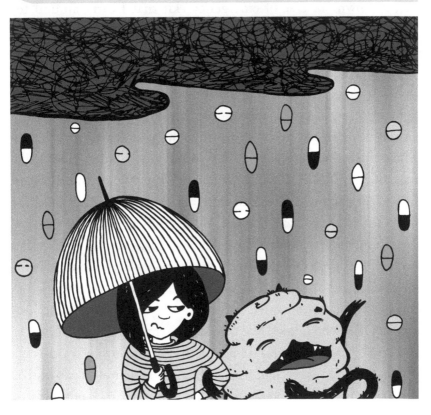

There are some things I have to have in my purse wherever I go, thanks to the anxiety monster. The stress ball that I stole from my kid's goodie bag, a candy, hand sanitizer (and this was important even before the global pandemic), and prescribed Clonazepam or as my doctor called them my emergency anxiety pills. I have those items with me even though my anxiety episodes have subsided considerably or even when I don't use these items as often as I used to. But each one of them is a key part of my safety net, my own "in case of emergency" kit that I carry around for peace of mind because I know those things work for me. However, to identify what worked for me took some time.

I get anxious while driving, particularly long distances. Traffic can be a trigger. I have had situations that even stopping on a red light or going over a bridge (more coming soon!) produces my anxiety. It is much better now, but I have the stress ball handy when I drive because it helps me to put my mind at ease. I like to squeeze it. After a while, when the toy is useless, I have to find a similar one to replace it. I always carry some candy for those times I feel dizzy. I know I don't suffer from any physical condition, and it's not like I need a little sugar rush to get back to normal, but probably the candy works as a placebo, and it helps me. The hand sanitizer that I always procure to be lavender, is something that I can smell and apparently nowadays it can also save my life (who knew?) Want to know why it works? All of those objects are distractors. Some people might prefer oils, or specific drinks, or listen to certain music. Some people only sleep with a particular weight blanket; others have found CBD products or herbal medicine very useful. I always have hemp oil, linden, and chamomile tea at home. What matters is that you find things that can help you momentarily. Again, it's like finding the right diet. Once you find the elements that work for you, everything will start flowing. Don't feel bad if you don't like what others like, or if something is working for someone else but is not working for you.

Let's get something out of the way and out of your mind right now. **I DO NOT** recommend alcohol or marihuana or any other recreational drug to be part of your "anxiety helpers crew." I will address alcohol consumption in a future chapter but marihuana or other drugs are not and have never been my weapons of choice and not my expertise. I won't be able to talk about this delicate subject which is a whole different kind of animal, so hopefully, you'll find additional literature to complement this book if you want to research substance abuse.

Nevertheless, "let's talk about meds, baby...." I can't stress this enough: You have to talk to your doctor. You need to understand that everyone is different and that our bodies respond differently to medications. I am usually in favor of medicine to get well when you need it. When I have a cold, for example, I don't try a million kinds of different teas and herbs first. I go straight to the over the counter medicine. Also, I have the fortune of having a brother who's a doctor so I can consult him at any time about any prescription I get if that is the case. However, when anxiety came to the picture, I created a HUGE resistance to medicine, but there is a story behind it.

My diagnosis came with an initial prescription of Zoloft, And I remember it working pretty well, and without any issues. At that time, I simultaneously started therapy after having understood that that was how you attack anxiety. Just a pill or any sole distractor won't make it go away. You have to assemble several things, like your own *Avengers* team of things that work in your favor, and this is a work in progress. One Avenger alone couldn't destroy *Thanos*. In your path to control your anxiety monster, you'll learn to recognize which *Avengers* you need and when to assemble them. Once you gather your win team you can start thinking about controlling your anxiety thinking long term instead of a momentary solution.

When I started meds and therapy, it was on my pre-motherhood years, so the anxiety monster behaved differently back then. After a few months, I was able to leave the pills and the therapy, always following my doctors' recommendations. Smooth and easy. Years passed, and as a mother, the anxiety monster came back in full force. I did what I knew. I went to the doctor again, and I was not scared about being prescribed another anxiety medication. The doctor prescribed me Celexa, and I decided to give it a try. Two days after I started the medicine, I got a massive panic attack in the middle of the night. I was sleeping peacefully when BOOM. Out of the blue, the hot flashes and then the dizziness. And It was so hard and sudden that I immediately thought it was related to my medication and not my anxiety. I felt that I was having one of those side effects that you never think they will happen to you. You know, those messages with the teeny-tiny letters on the box than you never read because hey, they won't happen to you. I was pretty sure that what I was experiencing was the Celexa side effects, and I only had a few minutes left to live. YES, it's that dramatic for us the anxious ones... and yes, it's exactly like in the movies when the character starts seeing flashes of his life in front of his eyes. My husband called 911 and I ended up in the ER (again, because this was not the first time) alone because hubby had to stay with kids, and also confused and terrified.

After they ran some tests, it turns out I was physically okay. It was anxiety. When these things happen, you feel incredibly embarrassed and guilty, thinking all of those resources, paramedics, ambulance, etc. were, after all, unnecessary. It's okay. You felt you were going to die, what were you supposed to do? What people need to understand is that the physical symptoms of anxiety are pretty scary, and they are real. I don't play around with these things. In terms of health issues, I seek treatment when I feel I need it despite what people say. I am a Momxious, I might go to the ER more often than a regular person but my peace of mind has no price, so better safe than sorry, and whoever wants to judge me, be my guest.

The doctor couldn't tell me if the Celexa was to blame or not for the episode. I remember he said he wouldn't think so because those medicines generally build up in your system and it takes several days to have any effect. Still, anyhow, he recommended suspending the medication until I could see my regular doctor. So, I did. More tests came back normal, but after this experience, however, I got utterly terrified of anxiety medication, and if the anxiety pills cause you anxiety, then what's the point? My monster was happy those days. I could feel it laughing at me and saying, "buckle up honey because there is no pill that is going to save you now."

There is also a predisposition to admit that you need medication help and moms take a lot of judgment on this one since the beginning. For example, it happens when people tell expectant mothers that taking the epidural is wrong because it somehow makes you less of a mother if you don't birth your child like in the cave times. Permission to roll your eyes granted! Technology and science help humanity, period. I am not less worthy because I take a shot or a pill to get better or to avoid pain. And having a mental illness is not different. If you need the medication, take it. Also, if you are sure you don't want to take this route, you don't have to, and that's fine. Everything is, after all, a choice. Herbs and natural aid are also available for you and as I said, do what works for you.

Don't feel embarrassed or pressured to use medicine or take herbs, or whatever route YOU think is the right one for you.

Let's go back to my story. I gave it a lot of thought and consulted my doctor again. I got the Clonazepam prescription, just in case of an emergency. The doctor told me that just having the meds in my purse could give me reassurance and that I might not even need them, but still, a bunch of questions and doubts came from the monster: "What if I get dizzy and sick again?" "What if I feel so good with the pill that I get addicted to it?" A few "what ifs" later, I was still not able to swallow a pill. Not even on one Thanksgiving night when I got another massive panic attack quite similar to the one I had when I started taking Celexa.

After months of trying different non-medication anxiety treatments, having good and bad days, there was an episode that made me change my mind. I was traveling from Vienna to Miami, a 10-hour flight with my husband and kids, and I decided to have some wine. I was exhausted. I hadn't slept well for days, and I thought that wine would help me to take a nap. Suddenly the monster appeared, and I thought I was dying. But I was on a plane! The combination of anxiety, exhaustion, and alcohol made me faint. It was a horrible experience that brought me back to my childhood dizziness spells. The loss of consciousness freaked me out in ways I can't describe. Everyone was so kind though, I got help, and I recovered. This kind of experience in public can make you feel embarrassed. It has something to do with showing vulnerability in front of others. Fainting can be terrifying because you wake up so confused and with a bunch of people looking at you. But it happens, and if it does, that's something else you have to cope with, along with other symptoms that you might experience.

Back at home in Jacksonville, because I had lost consciousness they ran again all sorts of tests. Everything came back normal, which is a good thing. Then why was I so angry? I enjoy traveling so much and I used to enjoy and relax while flying but the incident led me to develop a newfound fear of flying. Just like that, the monster took that away from me too. It's weird to understand, but sometimes when you have anxiety, you go to the doctor with the hopes that they tell you there is something physical that is causing you whatever it's you are feeling. It doesn't sound too good or at all coherent. Who would like to get a negative physical diagnosis? Us. Us anxious people, because our monster has convinced us that there is something wrong, or that someday something will be wrong and we should fear it. We want to find a more logical explanation of our symptoms because we think that is more acceptable than having anxiety. And we end up visiting the doctor more often than we should maybe because we know how to understand and undertake a physical illness but not a mental one.

I went back to therapy, but this is another story, and I guess it could be another book. Finding a therapist in the United States can become torture even when you have insurance. It's impossible to find someone soon, plus you need to find someone you can feel comfortable with, and the costs are absurd. Fortunately, there are more and more organizations that are addressing this issue, and nowadays, there is even online help available. But there is still a lot of work to do on this subject. Last year when I saw *Joker* I couldn't stop crying at the end of the movie because it made me think about this precise issue. As I said before, fiction sometimes helps us understand the complexity of our reality. The lack of mental health support in this country is a huge problem. Prevention is vital, but there's still a long road ahead of us to offer better tools, counseling, and to try to put a stop to unfortunate scenarios.

After the "plane incident," I created a new set of flying rules: No alcohol the night before, no drinking while aboard, and to take my emergency pill an hour before departure. Now there are times that I don't even have to take medicine. It all depends on the situation. The thing is that now I acknowledge that there are things out there that can help me and that I don't have to feel ashamed because I need them. Of course, ideally, someday I won't need anything. But while that day comes, if it happens, I need to cope with what I have in hand and what works for me. I am Nick Fury, and I will assemble my Avengers as I please when I need it. It gets easier when you find your own ways to feel better. To keep enjoying what you like. I was not going to allow the monster to terrify me so that I wouldn't travel anymore. It all starts with pure fear. So, before that happens, show the beast you have weapons, and if it wants to disrupt your life, you will not be afraid to use them.

 LESSON: You need resources to be able to control your anxiety monster and not the other way around. When you have identified your weapons don't be afraid to use them.

 TIPS:

- Be aware that what works for some won't work for others.
- Talk to your doctor or therapist about using a medication, if you are considering this route.
- Don't give up. There are tons of things out there on the market that you can use to cope with anxiety. Keep trying until you can assemble your own "in case of emergency" kit.

NOBODY IS GOING TO RESCUE YOU. YOU HAVE TO BE YOUR OWN HERO

"Nobody is gonna hit as hard as life, but it ain't how hard you can hit. It's how hard you can get hit and keep moving forward. It's how much you can take and keep moving forward. That's how winning is done."

-Rocky , Rocky Balboa

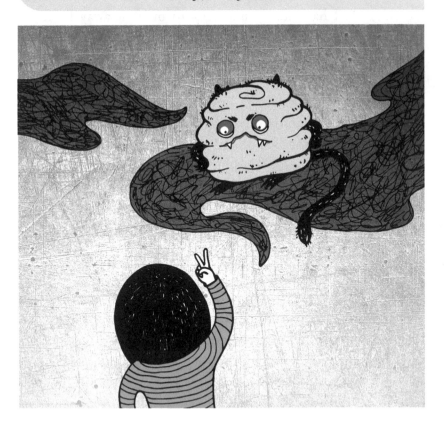

Travelling is one of the experiences I enjoy the most. Maybe because I spend most of the time alone at home, and even if it's a small getaway, it is my opportunity to connect with the outside world and enjoy life. However, since the Vienna incident, I noticed that I bring my monster as an extra passenger with me every place I go. It appears from the moment I start packing. It gets stronger the night before my trips and is because of it that sometimes I start thinking of airplanes or car accidents instead of the beautiful adventures I have ahead of me. It is extra heavy baggage, but I have slowly managed to move it away from my carry-on to cargo. Yes, it still travels with me, but it is not ruining my experiences like it used to.

My essentials for traveling are the destination, the circumstances, the activities, but mostly the company; I love traveling with my family. My kids have been going to different places since they were babies and they are perfect travelers right now. I think the experiences and the teachings behind any trip are unmeasurable, even when it is only a short camping trip an hour away. Of course, traveling with kids is different, but don't be scared of that possibility because it is marvelous for all. I enjoy spending time with my husband when we travel, we reconnect with each other once we change the scenery and we love to explore new cities together. We prefer to plan a trip over a gift on our birthdays or even for Christmas. Sometimes we plan trips with our friends and big camping getaways for celebrations and we have a great time with the people we love. Plus, both of us have our families abroad, so traveling is part of our lives. We have spent years visiting each other's countries of origin, which is an excellent experience for us as a family. Another good traveling experience for me is when my friends and I schedule a girl's trip. It doesn't happen often, but when we can pull it off is one of my favorite things to do.

It was all a bliss until the monster started appearing on my trips, then I got terrified of traveling. I started to develop fears that I didn't have before, and two, in particular, made my anxiety worse: A fear of flying and a fear of being separated from my family.

The Vienna incident was the start of these fears. From that moment, every single time I have an incoming flight, I replay the fainting episode in my head over and over. "Is this going to happen again?" that's the question I can't get out of my head. And just like that, something that I used to enjoy became a torture for me. I noticed how one fear could develop others and starts a chain reaction. Crowded places that I didn't mind before became a trap. The usual exhaustion after a day of walking in a new exciting city was the perfect candy for my monster, turning my experiences into complete anxiety episodes at the end of the day.

In an attempt to attack these new fears, I started to rely on others more and more. I was afraid of making decisions; I was in constant search for approval; I was even scared to drive long distances, and avoided certain activities. I lost control and let others run the show. I allowed the monster to be in charge of what I enjoyed, to take the wheel while I was riding shotgun. It was then when I started feeding my monster with the fear of being alone or traveling someplace without my family. I always thought that something terrible could happen to me, my kids, or my husband.

Eventually, my traveling fears transcended to my day to day life. I was always in search of another human being who could rescue me in every place I was. By then, I was still very private about my anxiety. I thought it was embarrassing if I contacted someone else saying I was having an anxiety episode. So, if I were running errands, I would check my surroundings and analyze who could help me if I fainted, or when the dizziness started I would frantically call my husband demanding that he would come to wherever I was. Most of the time, he was trying to calm me down over the phone. Other times my calls were so inconvenient that he would become frustrated. I don't blame him! Back then, I didn't know how to handle these situations, and he did not understand where my fears came from either. It was all a process for us as a couple and it takes time, love, and patience from both parts. It is important that we talk with our partner about our anxiety and that we are as crystal clear as possible, telling them what do we feel, and what do we expect. When another person gets frustrated with your symptoms don't take it personally. Remember that this is also confusing for them. If there is love it is possible and I can tell you it gets much better with time, but I understand, in the beginning, this could be chaotic and you can feel you are not supported. You feel isolated, and since you don't want to express yourself, you opt for remaining suffering in silence.

Everything changed for me when an opportunity presented itself, and I took it as a sign and a perfect setting to kick the monster's butt. While talking to one of my best friends, we were discussing how, as moms, we are always under pressure, and we forget to care about ourselves. We talked about our need to go away and started to plan a trip. You know how it is to plan a trip with your friends. There are weddings, pregnancies, babies, lactating periods, toddlers to run after, hectic schedules, or even a global pandemic, but something is most of the time always on the way. This time it felt like the gods had finally agreed to concede us the favor after years of planning such a getaway. We all needed the time for ourselves. For me, in particular, this came in a strange period of my life. I was battling with the new irrational fears, and I felt like I was losing control of everything in my life. There are perks of being a freelance writer. You can have your schedule and do things on your terms. But the financial instability can make you crazy. Also, at that moment, my self-esteem was not the greatest. However, the opportunity presented in front of my eyes, and I decided to jump on it.

We chose New York because we wanted to do something different than sipping margaritas on a beach, considering I live on the beach. Also, I was the only one in the group that had never been to New York. It also sounded so *Sex and the City*, of course without the sex but with the glam and scenery. So, I packed my bags, and I was very excited. Going away without my husband and kids meant not only that I was going to have time to be me, not a mom or a wife, nor I had to pack for and ensure the happiness of every single member of the family. This trip meant I had to take charge of my enjoyment as well as my anxiety. I was not going to be able to call my husband and demand him to rescue me. I had to deal with it by myself.

Of course, the monster appeared from time to time during the trip. Like at the end of *Wicked* (BTW, one of the most amazing things I have ever seen), when all the exhaustion of the day made me feel I was sinking into a hole and I almost ran away from the show. Gladly I didn't, and I finished it. Or when we were at the Statue of Liberty, and the crowd and narrow spaces were terrifying me, to the point I almost canceled the whole thing, but my friends encouraged me to keep going. We took beautiful pictures, and I felt so proud of myself for overcoming my fears. I didn't let the monster ruin the moment. But what saved me was the realization that I had to be my own hero.

First, I needed to speak more openly about my anxiety to the people I love. Because when it happens is also weird for them. They have no idea how to react or how to help you. You should not feel embarrassed. When I started to tell my friends and family about how I was feeling, all I found was support. As long as you make it clear that you are not trying to be fixed or rescued, you would be surprised by the amount of encouragement and love you get from others. The problem is when people feel they need to save you or when you make such demands. They can't make the monster disappear. Other people can't see your monster, and you need to be aware of this. It's like watching a child interacting with an imaginary friend. The most they can do is hold your hand, hug you, or tell you, "you can do this, I am here with you," or remind you to breathe. Tell them what you need from them, and they will be there for you. The people that are not willing to understand you and don't even try, the people that only give you judgments are not the people you need around you. They are toxic and you already know where to send those people.

I also decided, at that moment, to not hide on a shell. Hiding feeds the anxiety even more than having to experience it. Avoiding an activity is letting the monster grow bigger and stronger. Instead, you can choose to travel and live with the extra baggage, yes, but learn how to carry it so it won't drag you down.

Even if this sounds like a cliché, there is no better way to show yourself that you can deal with something than by dealing with it, the infamous "face your fears" thing. Don't try to fight fear. I kind of like the sensation now because I feel like life is presenting a test, an opportunity. When I am about to face a fear I apply a Yoda phrase: "No! Try not! Do or do not. There is no try." You might be missing amazing experiences just by avoiding a situation that you think will trigger your anxiety. And maybe it will trigger it, but trust me, you will feel incredibly accomplished, and there are significant lessons when you jump into your fear and realize that you can conquer it and that you are okay all by yourself.

If anxiety comes, let it be. You have been there before, and you know it won't go away just by wishing for it to disappear. We don't have magic wands or fairy godmothers. We also don't need another person to come and slay the dragon (I mean monster.) So, if it happens, let it happen. If you faint, or puke or pee (yes, it has happened to me), who cares! Please don't feel embarrassed, or weak, or less because you suffer from this and have a reaction to it. Those anxiety moments will happen, and they will pass. And you will go on with your life and the rest of the world too. There is no point in beating you up when these things happen. It's part of being human. You fall and clean yourself and move on. You keep on walking, learning every step of the way, becoming stronger every time you conquer an anxiety episode.

So, grab your cape Momxious because you are a superhero, go ahead and conquer the world, and be sure you can save yourself every single time you want to. You have the power, so own it!

 LESSON: People can't see or understand your anxiety, so don't expect others to save or fix you. Only you can do that by facing your fears. Believe in your power to rescue yourself.

 TIPS:

- Don't hide or avoid activities because of anxiety. Instead, prepare for those situations you might think will trigger them by knowing what works for you and having those 'weapons' handy.
- Don't feel embarrassed if you have a physical reaction to your anxiety. If it happens, know for sure the situation will pass. You have been there before, and life always goes on.
- Tell your loved ones how you feel and think of something reasonable you can ask from others in case of an anxiety episode. A hug, holding your hand, an encouraging word, a joke, singing along with you. The sky is the limit!

JUST BREATHE

"I know what I have to do now; I've got to keep breathing because
tomorrow the sun will rise. Who knows what the tide could bring?"
—Chuck Noland, Cast Away

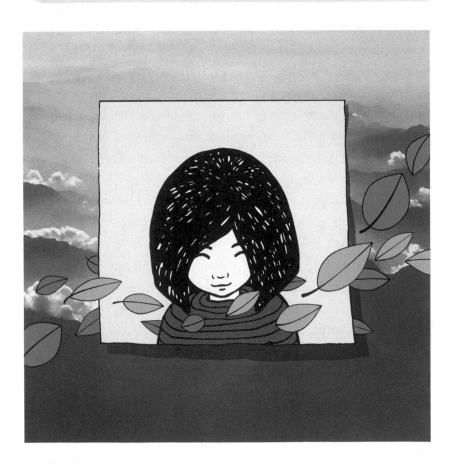

When the anxiety monster appears, it's like you get paralyzed and forget about the essential things, like breathing for example. A primary function necessary to live, something that usually we don't think about because it is mostly involuntary, but suddenly gets complicated when anxiety appears. I can recall one disturbing episode that happened to me while I was sleeping. I don't remember if I was dreaming about something in particular. All I know is that I woke up and had a terrifying panic attack; I was shaking, and I couldn't breathe! But then, and this happened in a matter of seconds, I started breathing frantically. One of the best friends of the anxiety monster is hyperventilation, this is when you breathe very fast causing a rapid reduction of carbon dioxide in your body, which leads to narrow the blood vessels that supply blood to the brain. This can produce one or several reactions such as dizziness, tingling in the lips, hands or feet, headache, weakness, fainting, and even seizures.

"How can a person have a panic attack while sleeping?" you may ask. I have no idea, but it happens. A few years ago, when I mentioned this episode to my therapist, he gave me a solution that changed my life. He said: "You need to remember to breathe." Then he explained a technique that works wonderfully for me — a breathing counting pattern technique called 4-4-4. You breathe in counting 4 seconds, then hold it for another 4 seconds, and slowly release the air counting another 4 seconds and repeat as many times it's necessary. Controlling your breathing can help you calm down, preventing hyperventilation hence other anxiety symptoms as well. I practice this as often as I can like Kegel exercises.

If this one doesn't seem appealing to you, let's try what every anxious person does. Google. But let's try it in another way, not in the "you have cancer and are going to die" mode. Don't Google symptoms, search for "breathing techniques" instead. Because if you get trapped in the Google symptoms search, it's like throwing your monster a birthday party with unlimited gifts. When you search for positive things and solutions, you may be surprised, but it's like opening a treasure box. You will be amazed to see how many theories and techniques about controlled breathing exist for example, and that can help you to recover in stressful situations in life, including anxiety and panic attacks. There is literature, a high number of YouTube explanatory videos, even gifs dedicated to this.

What you need to understand is simple, in life, sometimes we need to put a conscious effort into controlling our breathing. For example, when you are singing, running, swimming, etc., it means that you can learn to voluntarily manage your breathing and this is what you need to do when anxiety or panic attacks occur. Whenever the monster appears, breathing is the best weapon you have to kick the monster's and its friend's little butts. It would be best if you remember that you could control this function. Put this phrase everywhere, so you don't forget it: **JUST BREATHE.**

If you are driving, making a presentation, are in a plane or a restaurant, and the monster decides to appear out of nowhere, take that weapon out and attack him with a breathing technique. Memorize the phrase, repeat it, keep a note someplace you can easily see: JUST BREATHE. Whatever it takes to remind yourself that you can control it. I have put this phrase everywhere, and I am glad I have done this. I have a post-it inside my wallet and when I am out I know I have it there. I don't like tattoos personally but if I would do one this sentence would be it. My watch keeps telling me to breathe from time to time and I am grateful for that as well!

Remember, there is another breathe you need to take care of, but this one is less literal. I am talking about when you feel suffocated by people, work, or specific situations. For us, the anxious ones, it can be easy to get trapped into those without even realizing it, so it's essential to learn to identify those moments that you need to take some distance. Being afraid to say no or fearing being judged, it's when this usually happens. We can quickly get addicted to seeking reassurance, validation, and/or approval from others, so we often avoid confrontations and try to please other people first. Being aware of this and control it takes time and it's a process I have only mastered with time and practice. It can happen with your co-workers, your family, your friends, or even with a WhatsApp group, and you think that if you decide to take a break from those people, the relationship might break. Be sure this is not a Ross and Rachel situation; nothing will happen on this break if you need to take it. What I have learned is that sometimes taking a distance from someone, or a group can even be healthy and can also benefit your relationship with others. If you need to step aside to be alone or take your distance from certain people to be able to breathe, DO IT. Unapologetically. It doesn't have to be a prolonged break, sometimes just taking a walk will do. Leave that chat for a few days. You can always come back with a clearer head and understanding.

If you have to be more drastic, and you notice that a specific situation or person is draining you to the point that starts affecting your mental health, break it up completely. It takes courage, but you can do this. It often happens in work situations. Don't accept a job just because you need it or do something without passion; when you get trapped in a work environment that you don't enjoy or surround yourself with people that you can't stand, do yourself a favor and leave. It applies to romantic relationships too. Don't stay if you are suffering and your mental health is compromised. Drastic changes and decisions are hard to take; I get it. But you always have that choice. Find support with your family, use your creativity, pursue your passions. If you wake up every day and feel that going to your work is torture, or if you feel certain relationship is intolerable, this can be detrimental to your mental health and your anxiety can spiral out of control.

People can be overwhelming to an anxious person. Sometimes we need to be left alone. The important thing here is not to be rude. One thing is to cut toxic people from your life, and another one is to take distance from others when you need it, without hurting anybody's feelings. There are people in my life that I adore, but when I am anxious, I can't deal with them. So instead of engaging in an argument or force me to spend time or talk with them, I take distance for a while, deal with my issues, and then come back. Maybe you can try to explain to them that you need to take that distance, this is up to you, and you gage that one depending on the level of relationship and intimacy you have with the person or group. Also, it would help if you didn't withdraw completely. You can't become a hermit. We need each other to live and grow; we need to feel personal connections. Isolating yourself won't help you. It would be best if you nurture your relationships as well, and this is crucial to your anxiety coping.

Social anxiety is something I have dealt with from time to time. There are moments I just simply have to avoid people and gatherings. But I realized I was many times just making excuses. Sometimes parties or crowds can make you uncomfortable. And if you feel like that you don't have to force it. However, as I said before, we need each other. It became very clear for me just recently. I am in this very moment editing this book after a few months of being at home under the stay-at-home ordinance, thanks to the coronavirus threat. I got to admit, at the beginning of all of that I was not feeling uncomfortable. On the contrary, being at home is my comfort zone, so it was easy for me to cope with the situation initially. However, as time progressed and the situation started to unfold, things turned out to be more complicated. I had to use and test all of my methods to cope with anxiety more than anytime before. Suddenly I started thinking about how important it is for us to just be in contact with each other, gather, celebrate, or just talk. You don't know what you have until it's gone... We all realized that we need to socialize and have that human contact.

Another critical aspect is social media. If you need to unfollow people on social media, DO IT. There is nothing wrong with that. I have several friends I love and close to my heart, but their constant negativity online or overwhelming posts make my head spin. I snooze them, and it doesn't mean I don't love them. I also don't take it personally if someone decides to unfollow me. I can be overwhelming at times too. If people need to breathe from me, it's ok. I stand in a no-judgment zone. I have friends that have done it, and we still talk to each other.

We need to stop scrolling on our phones that often. We need to take a break from technology as well, which is why I strongly encourage you to detox from your electronic devices daily! Even if it is just for an hour. Maybe even for a day! It not only will liberate your time but also you will be able to breathe and get a better sense of reality. I am not against social media; I think it has its perks, and I love it! But since I started practicing this daily detox, I feel more relaxed. I usually select an hour in the morning and in the evening. It doesn't happen every day, but I try. It has changed my life. I am judging myself and others less. I stopped comparing my experiences with the ones portrayed out there where you don't know what is real and what isn't. I put effort into my creativity and consume less harmful and toxic content.

Sometimes what you need is just fresh air. Going out and spending time outdoors is a complete cure for the soul. Fresh air and nature are miracle workers. When you go out and start paying attention to your surroundings, you start appreciating other details in life. Most importantly, it can clear your head, give you new ideas, calm you down, see different perspectives. Give it a try when you need to breathe.

Breathing, in general, is essential for a mom. You NEED to have time for you to be you. It's normal to have those feelings when you don't want to be a mom or a wife, even if it's for a few hours. You need to have time to be yourself, to be the woman without a role in other people's life. I love to be a mom and can't imagine not being one. Feeling overwhelmed with the demands of motherhood doesn't make me love my kids less. If I have to breathe, I will, even if it is alone inside my closet, or locked in the bathroom. Sometimes you need a moment, and then you are fine.

Anxiety has caused me sometimes to get extremely angry at my kids. They frequently test out my levels of patience. I have sometimes snapped and yelled at them when they don't get ready on time for school after a bad night of sleep, or have arguments with my husband for many reasons like any average couple does. Still, due to my anxiety, sometimes I let my frustration take over my emotions. As a consequence, those interactions (normal in any family), resulted in me feeling exhausted, devastated, and burned out. Listen, your family is your family; they love you no matter what. You are the glue that holds everything together, and they need you. But they also understand (eventually) that you are not Wonder Woman (ok, you are.) Do whatever it takes to go out by yourself. Go for that girl's night out or trip. Don't skip the conference out of town. Find that friendly group on the MeetUp app if you don't know many people. Reach out, connect with others outside your family because you need to breathe from the mom/wife role. And when you lose your temper, don't be too hard on yourself. It happens. Breathe and move on.

My fellow mom, breathing, must become your first thought when you feel anxious, as it will help you find your center when your thermostat is all over the place. Because no matter what comes next, you need air to live, clean your soul (and lungs) of toxins and heavy burdens, no matter what obstacles and overwhelming situations, all you need to do is to keep breathing.

 LESSON: Controlled breathing techniques are the best weapon to be able to defeat the anxiety monster as it appears. Keep practicing them and set up breathing reminders wherever you go. Remember that breathing also means to set apart time for yourself, and this all requires your conscious effort, so don't give up, and JUST BREATHE.

 TIPS:
- Write the phrase JUST BREATHE in places that you can always see it. Let it be a reminder of a consciously focus when anxiety appears.
- Search the Internet about controlled breathing techniques. Try and adopt the ones that you like the most, and practice them wherever you can. Meditation and breathing techniques go hand by hand.
- Think of breathing as your weapon of choice to tackle a panic attack or anxiety episode.
- Remember that you also need to breathe (or break) from others. Don't hesitate to step aside and take your distance when you need to.
- Set time for yourself.
- Detox from your tech devices a few hours daily.
- Get outdoors. Nature is magic.

YOU ARE STRONGER THAN YOU BELIEVE

"Happiness can be found even in the darkest of times, if one only remembers to turn on the light."

–Dumbledore, Harry Potter

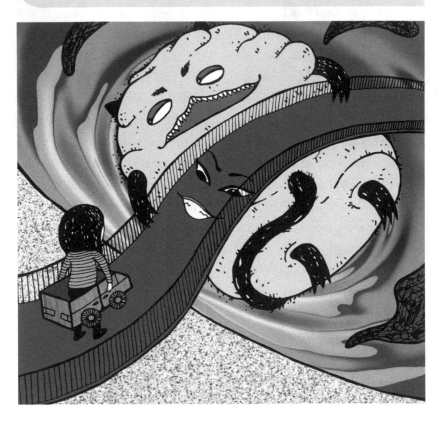

The anxiety monster tells you a lot of lies. But the one that I found most challenging to overcome is this one: YOU ARE WEAK. What a big fat lie! Along this process of re-discovery of being a mom battling anxiety, I've learned that a person that has to cope with a mental condition, or any health condition, in general, engage daily with unbelievable amounts of inner strength, that would not awaken if not because of said condition. It is as if somehow, anxiety has been a test all along for me to realize that I am the most powerful being, I know. That realization didn't come easily; because the lie that starts with the anxiety monster keeps being perpetuated by those around you and society.

There is a lot of stigma about mental illnesses. I have already talked about the extreme expectations that society puts on motherhood. Combine those two, and you get an explosion of shame over a mom that suffers from something like this. The monster already makes you feel that you are failing, that you are damaged, broken, that something is wrong with you, that you are having these emotions because you are weak. At the same time, people throw judgments at you, like if they have the authorization to evaluate you and give you a grade in an imaginary subject called "Mental Strength 101." The reality is that they have no clue about what they are saying. But I don't blame them either, is how they have learned to perceive others with this condition. Probably that single fact prompted me to start writing this book in the first place. I am a believer in change. It takes one idea to be able to inspire others, and I believe the stigma can change. Once I was feeling so low, so miserable and shameful because of the lie the monster made me think, that I thought I would never be able to recover or have a healthy life. Often, I was confronted by the judgment of people close to me by telling me things like: "Get over it," "Pull yourself together," or my favorite "It's all in your head." So, the more the monster appeared in my life, and the more I let the judgments affected me, the more I believed the "I am weak" lie, thus preventing me from actually trying to cope with anxiety. However, you can find enlightenment in your own anxiety experiences. For me, for example, I started to recognize my strength by overcoming those phobias the monster started bringing into my life.

Aside from the lies, the monster brings other uninvited guests to the party: Phobias. They appear unexpectedly, and you never see where they are coming from, or when they started to develop until one day you realize you have one and you can't get rid of it. The phobia is having the time of its life and doesn't care that the clock struck midnight, and it's time to go. She stays over and gets comfortable. Those strange fears start like a little snowball coming down the hill but quickly developing into monster phobias that menace all the progress you have made or, sometimes, becoming so powerful that it seems like they will crush you.

One day, I had a massive panic attack driving over a bridge, one that involved paramedics, sirens, and my terrified then seven-year-old girl in the back of my minivan. In the end, I recovered, managed to pick up my other kid, and went home to have some rest. Little did I know, this was the beginning of one of the strangest phobias my anxiety monster has brought along. That's how I welcomed **Gephyrophobia** into my life.

The fear of bridges characterizes Gephyrophobia, and its sufferers may avoid routes that will take them over **bridges**. The problem for me was that living in Jacksonville, Florida, (a city surrounded by water where you can't elude bridges,) this was the worse phobia I could get.

Many times, I found myself crying behind the wheel; I lost the count of how often I had to stop on the side of the road to find the courage to get over it. I tried to avoid certain roads, in particular, to avoid that single bridge, but I couldn't. I had to cross it almost every day because it was the only way of getting my kids to and from school. I started to get scared of driving. Some days it was unbearable and also challenging to talk about it. People didn't seem to understand anxiety, let alone that I was terrified of bridges.

Embarrassed and alone, somehow, I told myself I wasn't ready to let the anxiety monster and its new friend Gephyrophobia win.

A friend suggested that since I love fairy tales and fantasy, maybe I should try to imagine that across the bridge, I would find a fantastic realm to conquer. It was a matter of practicing that analogy combined with other techniques such as visualization for it to suddenly start working and killing my fear of crossing bridges. The realm, on the other side, was a colorful blend of sunshine, green grass, and happiness, and to get there I had no choice but to cross the bridge. I also started singing or joyfully screaming while I was passing. It was complicated, but soon I started noticing a significant change around the crossing-bridges-fear-pattern in my mind. I stopped going back to when I had that horrible panic attack and started creating new experiences to replace the horrific ones. Soon, I began liking the way I could see the sun rising and how the water sparkled every time I was on top of the bridge. I still wonder how I was never able to notice that before. I also discovered that the lovely sound of my boy's laughter and the music playing on the radio could give me the courage to cross the bridge. The fantasy analogy became a part of my reality, and crossing a bridge meant conquering new realms. It was a process, focusing on progress and repetition, which allowed me to see my inner strength. An opportunity to tell myself that I can conquer my fears, and it won't matter how ridiculous they sound to others.

What matters is that you are in this battle every day but you can also win it every day. And with anxiety, this is how you have to fight, becoming stronger and living each day at a time.

There are times, of course, when bridges make me feel anxious and sometimes afraid. I am aware that there are also tons of other phobias that the monster decides to bring along, but I don't believe in the lie anymore. I realized that I don't need to focus on what other people think. They cannot speak for me; they cannot grade me; their judgment is only a projection of their reality, not mine. I can choose to admit I am, in fact, strong and becoming stronger every single day. You have to learn to choose between believing the lie or finding your own path to unveil the truth. Sometimes, it takes to forcibly separate yourself from the negative experiences of the past, giving yourself the chance to create new experiences that show you how great you can be. Don't believe the monster, believe in yourself. You are not your phobias. You host the party of your life and let me tell you something; you can kick out those uninvited guests anytime because you have the right to do so and most importantly because you have the strength.

 LESSON: Sometimes, just by conquering a battle a day, you can uncover your inner strength. Let yourself win those little battles, and you will see how strong you really are. You'll be impressed!

 Tips:

- Try, try, and try some more. Don't give in to fears. It's ok if you don't get rid of the phobia at once. Just by trying and applying repetition, you can achieve progress.
- Use different techniques while battling a phobia. You can create analogies and use visualization to help you overcome certain

fear. Be ready with your favorite music or an app you can use (obviously not while driving) and try to create new memories that separate your thoughts from the past negative experiences creating new positive ones.

- Open your eyes and your mind. Sometimes fear doesn't let us experience something fully. It can make you blind. Look around you and focus on details that bring you joy, sounds, sights, tastes. Use all your senses!

TAKE IT ONE DAY AT A TIME

"What's comin' will come, an' we'll meet it when it does."
—**Rubeus Hagrid,** *Harry Potter*

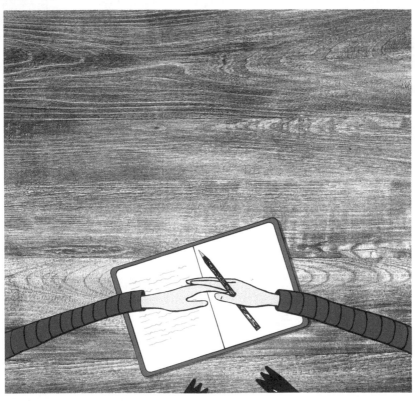

You are probably laughing at this one, aren't you? I know. The "one day at a time" approach for an anxious person and mom looks like something completely impossible to conceive, the biggest cliché you can find in self-help books. But I want to invite you to have an open mind. This approach is, in fact, beneficial and may help you immensely in coping daily with your anxiety.

This declaration is the same as asking you to honor the present instead of putting your energy, thoughts, and emotions on the past (the things that you can't change) or the future (the stuff you have no idea are going to happen or not) or both. Easier said than done, I know. And starting to live like this requires a lot of practice and patience. Some days you might be able to do it, some others not so much. Again, I invite you to at least try. Like one friend told me once. "Day one or one day. You choose."

Before I give you tips on how you can do it, I have to tell you how I started thinking like this. What comes next is very personal, and the first time I've come forward with this part of the story. But here we are, I want to be as honest as I can and show you how moms have vulnerable moments that by no means make us weaker or terrible, but can pull strength out that you could never have imagined you already had. I want to show you how we are human, and we make mistakes, but we can always make things right.

I love wine. It's one of my greatest guilty pleasures, besides coffee and soccer. It wasn't always that way. I think during my younger crazy years, I could drink everything else but wine or beer. One day you are young and drink whatever alcohol lands in front of you because you want "the buzz," and you can easily party all night long. Another day you are sipping wine at home watching a sunset because you enjoy the taste and just want to relax. So, for me, it was effortless to fit into the wine mommy culture right away. You know what I am talking about, we have all seen the memes, read the articles, or spoke with our friends, and even our kids, how mommy can't survive without wine or "mom juice." I even continue making jokes about it. If someone decides to do a study on how many preschoolers have written "wine" on the Mom's Favorite Drink category for those Mother's Day projects, I wouldn't be surprised if the answer is 90% of them.

Then yes, I was having a lovely relationship with wine and enjoying the pleasures of the occasional wine drinking. Until it stopped being occasional and became frequent, it happened quickly, almost unnoticeable, and the mommy wine culture contributed for me to think this was completely normal behavior. I was telling myself "every mom does it." I think the idea is that your consumption doesn't interfere with your life and affects you and those around you destructively or negatively. But in my case, it started becoming a bad habit.

The first sign that made me thought that the wine drinking was getting out of control was the harder and more frequent hangovers I started having. Not only was it more difficult for me to recover from them, but also, I noticed I was sometimes hangover during the week, something very unusual for me to experience. I didn't pay too much attention at first. I blamed aging. Until one day, things were scarier. My wine intake was causing a significant impact on my anxiety. Yes, I was using the mom wine culture to justify my wine drinking, not only to normalize the situation but also as a magic relief for my anxiety. I won't lie; a glass of wine takes the edge almost immediately for me. But If I get too much of it, which started to happen more often, I am a mess, and my anxiety is THE WORSE. I can't emphasize this enough. MY WORST ANXIETY EPISODES HAVE HAPPENED AFTER CONSUMING MORE ALCOHOL THAN I SHOULD HAVE. After a binging wine session, my anxiety is almost unbearable, and

I can't even get out of bed, I am terrified and sick. I shake and feel I will faint at any time. When this happens, I can see my monster right there next to me laughing and telling me, "I told you so," with a big smile on its face.

One morning I was driving my kids to school. The night before I had had some wine. I had a terrible headache when I woke up and felt week and overall restless. I thought maybe I just needed to sleep some more, so I planned to come back home and have some needed rest. However, things turned out worse. When I started to drive, I had a massive panic attack while at a red light. I parked the car and recovered from it, but once I started driving again, the anxiety came back. I had to stop several times to cope with the anxiety I was experiencing, enhanced by the physical consequences of alcohol consumption the night before. I felt dizzy, I was shaking, obviously dehydrated, and feeling terrible because the only thing I wanted was to get my kids to school safely. I decided to call a friend to pick up my kids and take them to school. After a few minutes of recovering alone, crying uncontrollably in my car, I was able to go back home. As I was lying down in bed later that day, I was struggling with the question, "what am I doing to myself and my family?" Yes, it crossed my mind that I might be an alcoholic and this thought terrified me. Once you realize that your actions are affecting you and your family you have to take action. After that episode, I did my best to change the behavior, and I got to say things got much better. But then I noticed that the situation was somehow repeating on some weekends with me having wine on Friday night and having active panic attacks the days after.

I fell into a dark circle of guilt and anxiety that I tried my best to cover from everyone I knew, including my own family until something MAJOR happened. Something that struck me harder than if a thousand bricks had fallen on my chest. While I was picking my daughter's mess in her room, a paper on the floor caught my attention. I read it once. "I wish my mom wouldn't like wine that much!" Nothing in my life has hurt me more than this. And this was the wake-up call I needed.

I was so angry at myself because I made this situation happen. I turned a bad habit into a potential danger. What's worse, I used my anxiety to justify my irrational and destructive behavior. As a mom, there is nothing worse than breaking your kid's heart. I needed to fix this —this time, I had to do something more permanent. I knew I had the strength, and mostly, I had a significant reason to get rid of that bad habit. Things were not so out of control yet, but I knew that if I wouldn't put limits and change, I was on the road to disaster. I understand that parents, one way or the other, somehow mess up from time to time, and this is a fact. We can't be perfect because we are still human beings in constant self-discovery, we keep growing despite how old we are, and in that process, we can hurt our kids and sometimes we won't even be able to notice it. However, when we do, and we have the conviction that we can change, we can take action. There are just two choices; we can either dwell on the situation or try to fix it. I chose the second option. Accepting you are not a perfect mom is the first step. If it helps, you should scream it out loud right now: I AM NOT A PERFECT MOM!!! It feels good, doesn't it? And now let me tell you, YOU DON'T HAVE TO BE.

So, this is what I did. To change my behavior, I had to change my mentality, surrender, and then change habits. But here is the secret, I realized that I had to take the one day at a time approach. Thinking about long term results was not doing anything for me but giving me more anxiety. I decided to add the word TODAY to common sentences as I was planning my days. I was telling myself things like: "Today, I will go to the gym." "I won't drink wine today." "Today, I am really anxious; I will lay down and take it easy." "Today it's a beautiful day to go for a run." "Today I am going to start reading that book I have on the shelf."

While I was doing this, I also grabbed my set of beliefs and put them to work. Call it God, Universe, Supreme Power, even The Force. If you believe in something external out there, which is my belief, it exists; this is the time to call it into action. At this time, I worked so hard to feel connected to that spiritual power, praying, meditating, and reading about how you can ask help from the universe. I soon started feeling better, I released the guilt, and felt supported and guided, but taking all one day at a time. I discovered that the art of surrender is the most beautiful thing in the world.

Soon I started noticing significant changes. I was going to the gym more often during the mornings. I liked it because it filled me up with energy and I felt healthier. Remembering I had a spinning class the next day or a planned run for the morning, made me put down the glass for days without even thinking about it. The new healthier habits helped me to enjoy wine responsibly and now I don't even consider this an issue nor I feel the necessity of drink wine to ease my anxiety. I started feeling much better overall. Trust me, life is not perfect, there are still days that I make mistakes. I am human, and my bad habits can come back I am aware of that. But I understand that with consistency and awareness, things can get better. I learned to know my limits and realize when I am crossing the line or I am about to. I started to listen to my body and my soul and forgive myself every time I made a mistake to move on. However, getting into a better, healthier, and more enjoyable relationship with wine taught me that we can change big things, starting with just one step in the present. To have that future you dream of, you have to have a better now because those steps you are taking will take you where you want to be. You can't change the past, but you can take action in the present.

I started using this approach for everything after, particularly with things that affected my anxiety. Planning on a short-term basis helped me tremendously, and I was able to achieve more. I became more productive because just taking it one day at a time, immediately took away the tension from those big future expectations. For example, I stopped having New Year's resolutions. I realized they create more anxiety because you put so much pressure into achieving things that you don't have. Instead, now I make a list of New Year's instant actions that I can make to have the great year I want to live. The "I want to go down three sizes by April" became, "I am going to move or exercise for 30 minutes daily and eat cleaner foods starting today." Instead of "I will publish a book by October," I say, "I am separating one hour daily to write." And guess what?, the results are even more significant because I am focusing on my daily achievements, enjoying the steps along the way instead of future tripping and failing constantly. It has also helped me with overthinking and with other habits that I want to change. When I have those "fail" days, I can move on faster and correct what I need to achieve progress. Of course, I have long term plans and big future objectives, but they are not the center of attention anymore.

Achieving small daily things resulted in significant accomplishments later on, and having the confidence that I was able to improve helped me to see problems differently. There are always solutions and guidance daily. This approach enabled me to finish and publish two books, started and finished the one you are reading right now, got healthier, happier, and with much less anxiety all in one year. For example, I have no idea how much I weigh, but I feel good about myself and with my choices. And

I continue enjoying wine, a chocolate cake, or even occasional comfort foods, knowing that moderation and self-control are entirely achievable, stopping the monster to influence my choices.

The whole key to this approach is the following. You have to forgive yourself for your mistakes daily and make a conscious decision to move on, no matter what happened or what it takes. Whatever goes wrong during a day, you have to forgive yourself, make a move, and let it go. Also, it is about celebrating your small daily victories. Please pay attention to the road because it's all about the journey and not the destination. There is a great British rom-com I recommend you to watch that speaks about this. If you have the chance to watch *About Time*, do it, you'll love it!

After all, if you enjoy the blessing of a new day, this approach will help you to appreciate that your life is giving you a unique opportunity to grow every single morning, a chance to keep moving forward and be a better human. Daily. There is no bigger miracle than that.

 LESSON: Every day is a new opportunity to be better, to change those things that are pulling you down, and grow. Be aware that you have the chance of having the kind of day you want and that little daily achievements can result in substantial life accomplishments in the long run.

 TIPS:
- Have a journal. I took this advice from several authors and experts, and it's a miracle worker ritual. It takes just a few minutes in the morning and before bedtime. Feel free to be creative on how to use your journal, but here is an idea. I have developed a 3-step journaling routine with some basics. I believe that the key is not

only about what you write but writing from a place of love. So to put me on that state I pray and meditate for a few minutes then I answer some specific questions in my journal such as "how I want to feel today?" "5 things that I am grateful for are..." among other things. If you want to get deeper into my method I host journaling webinars all the time and my Momxious Journaling Method is available on my website, with templates and things you can use. You can also find effective journaling by describing your day ahead imagining how good is going to be or put things that you are expecting to happen or actions you are willing to take today toward one of your dreams.

- End the day exploring in your journal what was great about it and how it could have been better.
- Write down positive affirmations and read them every morning and night. There are tons online, or you can create your own. Aside from the 18 declarations in this book and that you can use daily, I am giving you this one: **Anxiety doesn't define me. I can forgive my past, honor my present, and allow the future to happen. I am safe, and every day I am feeling better. I love my imperfections. I am grateful for my mistakes because they are helping me to be aware of things I need to transform to feel better.**
- Write down the declarations of this manifesto and read them out loud. Put post-it notes around your house, or your computer, have them handy on your phone. When you feel anxious, reread them.
- Don't spend much time on future or past tripping. You are not a *Dark* character. Instead, try to think about the actions you can make right now to achieve or change something you want. But if you do future tripping, concentrate on how it makes you feel, imagine achieving something you dream as if you are already there. Let your imagination put you in a place of peace and

comfort. Don't focus on what you don't have yet, but in what can you do now that will take you there. Let the emotions inspire you to take action.

LEARN FROM YOUR GOOD DAYS

"My Mama always said, 'Life was like a box of chocolates; you never know what you're gonna get.'"

— Forrest, Forrest Gump

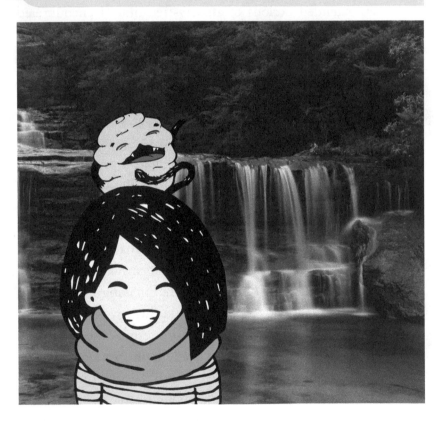

The good thing about being more present, taking it one day at a time is that you can identify your progress and your failures in more specific ways. You also start having more good days than bad days. It didn't happen overnight for me. But yes, once I got a commitment with myself to being more aware of my current situation, I started turning my relationship with the monster around as well. Soon I noticed how many good days were turning into more extended periods of anxiety-free time. I encountered myself enjoying life fearlessly, even forgetting about that nasty creature. I was more present, vibrant, and focused. More pleased with life and eager to explore my purpose in the world. However, this monster is a tricky one. Of course, after too many of those good days, I found myself wondering about the monster and asking myself: "where did it go?" "This is too good to be true," as if I would miss it. I was expecting it to appear at any moment, wondering when it would come back to rain on my parade, subconsciously calling it again into my life.

The monster has that ability; it can be active even in its absence, but I discovered that this is a power that only I can give it. Hence I can also take it away. How? The answer sounds easy; however, it takes practice. Once I mastered making it one day at a time, I pushed the concept even a little further, particularly in those good days. When you are having one of those, you need to take advantage of them to train your brain to be present not only with the "today" concept but also with the "right in this very moment" one. Although this is entirely achievable, it's incredibly complicated for an anxious person. But you can do it. I promise you. And it doesn't have to be all the time; if you learn to do this as much as you can, it will help you even if it's sporadically. What happened to me is that the good days started to become great teachers, and living in the present taught me more about the meaning of happiness and how to embrace my emotions. Although this is not a permanent situation, especially when you live with anxiety, that is why I value those good days and learn from them because they always bring something new to the table.

I know, for us, the anxious ones, it's difficult not to think about the future, immediate and long term, or to have fixations on past events and experiences. We wish we could have a magic device handy so we can see through it and get reassurance for the future. Or perhaps a magic trick that could erase the feelings that trouble us when we can't let things go. I see now that living that way would only bring me more anxiety. But I am also aware that living permanently in the now is also very hard. Somehow, I needed to come up with a plan to put in action when my mind decided to travel along time, especially when I was having those good days because mind time traveling can be an open invitation for the monster to appear. So, I created a method, a guide for redirecting my thoughts, which I've called "The Comeback Method." You can use this whether you are having a good or a bad day (however, in bad days, the process is different, and I will address that in the next chapter, so let's focus on the good days for now.)

Let's say you are having a great day, and sudden thoughts start attacking you. And because you know your feelings are uncomfortable you are thinking about the monster, expecting it to appear. You need to remember that you give the power to your thoughts. The way you can identify if the energy is negative or positive is by knowing how are you feeling. If you provide the wrong power to the thought, your happy and calm day can turn dark. So, before this happens, **"come back."**

This is an example of how usually the whole thing unfolds: You are enjoying yourself, and you are monster-free. Then out of nowhere, you get a thought. Maybe you are thinking about something that you want, but you don't have yet, or something that has hurt you, or a situation that you want to get resolved, but you don't have a solution just yet. You start feeling discomfort, a pressure. The monster is not there yet; however, you feel it's coming; you feel it's presence, like Luke Skywalker sensing his father approaching, and this is the moment when you need to go back (before The Imperial March starts playing in your head.) Quickly replace the thought with something that has made this day a great one. Come back to the present time consciously. Think in terms of THIS EXACT MOMENT. What are you currently enjoying out of your life? What is great at this very exact moment? What do you appreciate the most right now? What are the things that are working in your life as you breathe? Also, you can use visualization, picture your children's smiles, that's always an easy comeback moment if they are not the ones causing you anxiety at the moment!

Another thing you can use to come back is a happy memory, if you are a mind time wanderer, like me. And I know that I have advised you to avoid this but when it happens is better that your mind time travel be a positive experience. So, in these cases, permit yourself to "go back" to "come back," like *Marty McFly*, who had to travel to the past to fix the present, sometimes it helps if you don't go there to dwell on the what happened. Or, even better like the characters of *Inside Out*, let your "Joy" put a happy memory in your head. Think of a memory of a past great day, a significant achievement that made you feel good, the moment you saw your child for the first time (that's also a good one,) think of the butterflies you felt when you fell in love, or about that dream you had the other night, and you can't stop thinking and smiling about. The key to the comeback method is that you instantly feel good, if you are feeling good it means the thought brings you back to the peaceful and calm setting and emotions.

Meditation is another resource to come back. As I have explained before, there are many approaches to meditation. I have found that listening to mantras during my meditation practice can change my energy instantly. There is a mantra that I have handy when I feel a slight negative thought or emotion: "Ek Ong Kar Sat Gur Prasad" often used to reverse negative to positive. Type this one on YouTube or Spotify, and you will find several versions of music with this particular mantra. When I feel stuck, sometimes, I just take my dog out for a walk, put my headphones, and listen to this mantra for at least 10 minutes.

If I feel more energetic, I also use running to come back. Or if I am in the car and nothing of the above helps, just putting music out loud works wonders. You can even find your own come back methods; the important thing is that you can identify what gets you back into feeling good and use it as much as you can.

Once you are again in a happy state, you need to train yourself to think about the future and the past in different ways. When you plan your future, don't focus on what you don't have yet, focus on the actions you are taking right now to get where you want to be. In this way, you can be more proactive. If you fixate on a past event and it's making you uncomfortable, you need to realize that when your mind goes there, you are just a mere observer. The difference between you and *Marty McFly* is that you don't have a DeLorean Time Machine, so you can't change anything there. What happened, happened. So, come back to today and ask yourself what the lesson behind that thing you are obsessing about is? And how you can apply that lesson today IN THIS EXACT MOMENT. If you fought with someone, or if you made a mistake, there is nothing you can do there at that time. Obsessing about what happened won't change what happened, but certainly, you can take the lesson, forgive, and move on, and maybe fix things in the present.

I also want to invite you to think about the term happiness and what it means for you. People tend to believe that a good day means to be happy all day, but then, what does it really mean to be happy? I will explain why this is very important. "How can I expect to be happy all the time? It's impossible!" I get it. We are humans, complex beings with all sorts of emotions. However, emotions are momentary. I stopped seeing happiness as pure emotion, but as a general, a more permanent state of mind, and that should be the goal. If I feel happy with my life, other emotions that are momentary will not affect that general, more permanent state of mind. They influence the moment, but that's all. For me, excitement, fun, pleasure, calm, sadness, anguish, despair, anger are emotions, reactions to the day to day life, and they are momentary. They last for a few minutes, hours even. But to be happy or unhappy have a more general connotation. I can be overall satisfied with my life, enjoy my journey, what I do, my choices, but someday something happened to me that made me react with a particular emotion that makes me momentarily "something." For example, if I am angry at someone that I just disagreed with it doesn't mean that I am unhappy with my life.

Anger takes a moment. Then I use the comeback method. I probably won't come back to be exited or exhilarated right away, but when I come back, I can be at least more serene, and that's enough to remember that I am happy with my life. All it takes is to replace the thought to replace the emotion. And there is where I found balance. Life is about the enjoyment of it, disregarding the momentary emotion. It took me time to realize that I love my life, and I am happy with my experiences, with all that it entails, positive and negative momentary emotions, because all made me grow and learn. If I am grieving, of course, I am not jumping and dancing because my human nature needs me to process the loss, and for that, I need to experience sadness first. But I can slowly come back, knowing that overall, I am happy with my life and for sure someday again when the grief is gone, and the sadness overcame, I can still be excited and exhilarated.

If I am having a good day, and I feel a momentary negative emotion, I understand it is my choice to engage or not with what is causing it. Frustration, anger, melancholy are triggers for me. The instant I feel those things, I apply the "Comeback" method. If I don't engage, the monster will retract.

Another important lesson all of this has taught me is that I am the ONLY PERSON responsible for my happiness. Also, I am not responsible for anybody else's one, including my kids and my husband, the closest to whom I share my life. You can't make a person happy, and another person can't make you happy; this is a personal path. Trying to change other people or "fix them" won't make them happy like other people trying to change you or "fix you" won't make you happy —the moment I realized that, I started to look for and find my own happiness. And here I am. It is discovering that by trying to be more present, positively dealing with momentary emotions, I can live better and enjoy my overall happy life, and this was a lesson that I learned only by observing and absorbing my good days.

In a previous chapter, I told you about the habit of journaling; make this a priority in your life because this will help you a lot with planning your days and keep your feet and mind on the present. Also, when you read your past entries, it's an opportunity to revisit the lessons learned. If you start the day with a conscious desire to have a great day, the possibility that the day will indeed be great is so much higher. Another benefit is that you will, be little by little, more aware of the things that make you feel good instead of focusing on the absences and the monster. You will also start seeing more things to be thankful in your life. You begin to make peace with who you are and the situations that surround you, focusing on creating solutions instead of listing the problems. And the most important thing. Know and believe that you are deserver of good days and treasure and enjoy them to the fullest!

 LESSON: Enjoy the good days and train yourself to be as present as you can be, knowing that the future and the past are times that you have no control over. Focus on your feeling-good state and emotions, and come back to it as needed.

 TIPS:
- Don't forget to journal every day.
- Remember the comeback method by using a resource that works better for you or fits your particular situation (happy memory, meditation, activity, music...The sky is the limit!)
- Feel and believe that you are worthy of good things and feelings, and let yourself enjoy the good days. Notice the greatness around your life, and be more thankful for these moments.

RESPECT YOUR BAD DAYS

"I will not say: do not weep; for not all tears are an evil."
—**Gandalf the Grey, *The Lord of The Rings***

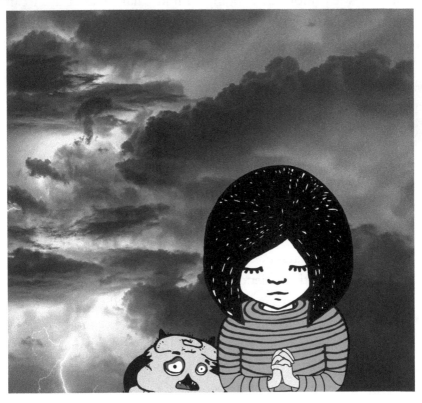

Even though the purpose is to always come back to the balanced overall happy state, there are dark days. I believe everyone has those and whoever says they don't they are lying. We are human, and as such, we are dealing with all sorts of experiences and emotions. Yes, I agree that the control of such feelings and experiences is different for everyone and that for some of us, sometimes it is more challenging to find balance, after all. I can repeat the following sentence thousands of times, and I encourage you to do the same. If you happen to fall in the category of those who take longer or need a more significant effort for controlling your emotions, know that it DOESN'T mean that you are a weak person or weaker than others. Your experiences are only yours, and your inner strength doesn't need validation, nor your conditions in life determine it.

Now that we got that out of the way let's talk about the dark days. The monster is there, and there is nothing that makes it go away. My dark days are usually the days that I can barely move. I want to lie down and do nothing. I can't even shower. Everything and everybody irritates me. As I have mentioned before, sometimes anxiety invites other friends to the party, like depression, for example. So, in my case, in those dark days, I usually have no energy, sometimes I cry, sometimes I don't. Overall, I feel unmotivated. It's a very uncomfortable feeling, and often, we feel ashamed to feel like this. It's hard to explain this sensation to others, and we are scared to show this side of us because we think we'll get judged. The thing is that no matter what, life goes on and the world doesn't stop because you have a bad day. You still have so many things to do, responsibilities, work, children, you name it. Before my self-exploration journey, I just tried to seclude myself as much as I could. But since life had to go on, I felt that in such cases, I had no choice but to let the monster follow me wherever I went. "Fake it until you make it" through the day seemed like a perfect motto.

Things changed, fortunately. And there was an experience for me that showed me this clearly. It happened not too long ago, over family vacations at Whistler, Canada. I enjoyed the trip, the snow, the mountains, the skiing (even though I suck!), it was a fantastic trip. The night before leaving while we were packing, I broke my "no drinking" rule and had a few more glasses of champagne than I should have. I got carried away, and even when I knew it was a mistake, I ignored my instincts. The next morning, with the travel ahead, getting the kids ready, and with a bad hangover, my anxiety went through the roof! No coming back method worked, but I still needed to travel from Whistler to Jacksonville, Florida, with kids. It meant a two-hour car ride, two planes to catch, and a new car ride home. I am fortunate that my kids are excellent travelers. Also, my husband already knows that traveling makes me anxious, so he takes charge. We have been traveling with the kids since they were babies, so, they are pretty comfortable with long traveling, (also, thanks to Steve Jobs for your inventions, parents around the globe are forever grateful.) Still, long travels are stressful, no matter what. I was on the bus ride to the airport, trying not to focus on my already almost unmanageable dizziness. Since I needed a distraction, I turned to Facebook (here I have to thank you, Mark, even though I have a love and hate relationship with your invention.) I have subscribed to a couple of anxiety support groups there, which I find can be useful and evil. Sometimes it helps you to vent because you know that most likely, there won't be any judgments. Those groups have precise rules and are regulated. But other times, you feel extremely overwhelmed with the posts. Here I am going to take advantage of the subject to make a side note. Please DON'T use these support groups for medical advice —just DON'T. You may put your life at risk. They work wonderfully as support, or if you have to vent, but please always seek a doctor's opinion in terms of medication or any other medical information you request.

Let's continue with my story. That day I thought posting something there would help me, or at least I could talk to people that would understand what I was feeling. I posted that I was extremely anxious and that I had this trip ahead of me, and I was terrified. I found a lot of support, and people started replying and giving me courage and advice. There was one comment that stuck on me. A person said this: "This day will happen no matter what. And will end no matter what. Try your best, and know it will be over." Little did that person know that this sentence not only kept me going through the day but also, changed me forever.

The day went through as that person described. It was that simple now in retrospect. The day happened! I got dizzy; I cried, I was anxious, and I felt terrible. But I still had to do it. And indeed, it ended. At the moment, it wasn't that simple, though. I went through the day, repeating that sentence in my mind like a mantra. And I did my best. I tried to drink water, went through my breathing exercises, tried to sleep when I could, and for moments, I was fine, others I wanted to find a hole to drag me down. The hours seemed eternal, but I kept repeating the sentence emphasizing the part that it was going to be over at some point. Until I was finally home, the kids went to sleep, and I was trying to do the same, but I stayed awake in my bed for a little while, silently thanking that person that I didn't know but who with a single sentence held my hand through the dark day. And I slept, and it was over.

Dark days will happen. They are part of this. Now when I have one, my comeback method consists of me repeating that only sentence over and over in my head or even out loud. Because I know that in these moments there is not happy memory, song, or thought that I could use to come back. The sentence helps me to move on the day hour by hour. Step by step. Task by task.

So ok, let's say I am so anxious and dizzy, but I still need to take the kids to school. If I feel so bad that I can't drive, I call an Uber. Hold on; I have no money to spend on that! Then let's take the courage and drive. Oh, but I am feeling so anxious in the middle of the road, it's okay, I can stop. Nothing will happen if the kids are a few minutes late. Later I come back home, and the house is a mess, and all I want is to take a long nap, then I am unapologetic about it and take the needed rest if I have to. The house can be like that for an extra day. Who cares? Queen Elizabeth is not coming to visit today anyway! Plus, I don't owe anybody explanations on how I am feeling. I need to go through the day. So, if you have to cancel that appointment, take that day off, call for help, or if you really can't avoid the day like in my back-home trip, go through it little by little —one task after the other. Sure, the monster will be there. Annoying you, telling you, "You can't get rid of me. I told you so!" You are allowed to be angry at it. Scream at it if you need to. Anger can be a little better than fear. It will become a momentary emotion, and then you can slowly come back to calm. Don't expect that from an extremely intense negative emotion, you will jump back on the excitement train right away. It has to be slowly, "Des-pa-ci-to" (Thank you, Luis Fonsi!)

Whether it's a good or a bad day think about your thoughts this way: each one can generate an emotion that will determine your balance. If it's a positive emotion, cultivate that thought. If it's a negative one, try your best to replace it. Imagine that your mind is a vast library, in which each book is a thought. And you are picking them one after another; they ignite your imagination and create a chain reaction that can make you feel good or bad. If the feeling is terrible, then change your book. You can do it.

You can control it. Change the book as many times is necessary. And if you think you made your best effort and still feel bad, then do nothing at all. **Sometimes to DO NOTHING is doing SOMETHING.** If there is no energy, no imagination, nothing you can do, just rest.

Allow yourself those moments of not putting effort into anything whatsoever. If you need to hire help with your kids, do it. Or if you need to recruit a friend to help you, do it. Surround yourself with people that can come to you in those dark days. I understand you might want to be alone, but if things get so overwhelming that you can't function on your own, ask for help. What matters is that if you need to, you have to put your mind and body to rest. The other day someone told me that the way up is not a straight line. I would add to that sentence, it's also not a lonely ride. We need people to push us, held us, or be there next to us for company.

Those days will happen, that is a life fact. Just remember, they will be over no matter what. I am going to give you another piece of advice, a method that works for me. Think about the nighttime like your reset chance, when your system is just stuck or have crushed. It's the opportunity to recharge. Before going to bed, take your journal, write your intention of having a good rest that night. And also, your purpose of having a good day once you wake up. Then you can take a warm shower and imagine all the negativity washing away. This tactic has made my nights more enjoyable, so much than when I have one of those bad days, I am looking forward to it because the night represents the end of it —my chance, to go away for a few hours and let my mind wander. My periods of insomnia have also been considerably reduced just by following that pattern during nights. When I write things down is like putting my intentions to the universe and surrender to the power beyond. The beauty of life is that if we are allowed to have another day, you can start all over again.

As I write this chapter, I am thinking again about the person that told me that crucial sentence and its impact on my life. Even in dark moments, you are still learning, so open your heart for new lessons even when there are clouds in the sky. Always do your best and nothing more. However, and this is very important, if the next day the darkness still there and the monster is refusing to leave, you have to take more drastic measures to get out of that state of mind. Back to back dark days can swallow you into a more dismal vicious cycle that can lead you to an overall unhappy territory, and that's how you feed your monster. Remember, you can come back, you have tools and people that can help you. So, repeat the methods as often as necessary and have faith in yourself and your ability to find the light. Allow yourself a day or two to come back to a more stable state, to a happier you. Slowly. Probably the next day won't be completely dark; it can be cloudy with a chance of rain, but you are going to be on your way to finding the sun again because it's always there regardless. You can find it, and when you do, soak up on that light. Remember that you overcame the dark day, and now you are enjoying the sun. You can do this as many times as you wish. So, in the end, those dark days are lessons. Respect them, don't fear them. Let them be because they teach you and test your strength. But don't let them stay.

 LESSON: Dark days will happen, and they don't mean you are weak. See them as an opportunity to practice resilience. Try your best, respect them, but don't fear them, and no matter what, don't let them stay. Remember, the day will be over, no matter what.

TIPS:

- Keep trying the comeback method and go through the day one task at a time.
- Replace the thought, always looking for something that makes you feel better.
- Don't force yourself into situations to find validation or because you think you have no choice.
- Rest your mind and body if needed.
- Write your intentions in your journal. Use the night as your reset button and repeat as needed.

FORGIVE AND FORGET

"The past can hurt. But the way I see it, you can either run from it or learn from it."

—Rafiki, The Lion King

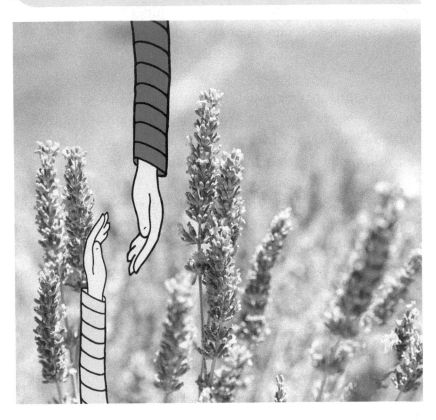

There is one thing that triggered my anxiety that my monster loved the most: my inability to let things go, especially when it had to do with relationships with other people. I was often getting stuck with the things I couldn't let go of. Discussions, disagreements, the judgment of others or things people said that bothered me are some of the things that have caused me mayor levels of anxiety in my life. Why? Because I wasn't able to forgive and forget, meaning I wasn't able to let things go. Little by little, I was engraving my mind and my soul with labels, a product of the things that bothered me and that I seemed not to be able to get resolved. When you don't "let go," you soon find yourself in a labyrinth. You are desperate to get out, but all you see around is big walls. Regret, pain, words left unsaid, actions you didn't take, but you should've, or moves that you made or words that you said and you shouldn't have, built those walls, and you can't seem to escape those things simply because you don't let them go.

My anxiety used to get heavily triggered when those situations happened to me. But on my journey to recover, I discovered an enormous lesson about this. Letting go is an art and you can learn to master it. Trust me, once you do it, you can be singing "Let It Go" from the top of your lungs and with a completely different meaning this time, plus your kids are going to love it! (Even better if you have an Elsa wig on.)

The inability of not letting things go, like any other thing that affects you and put you in sync with negative emotions usually come from past experiences that somehow got imprinted by your 'Ego.' I don't want to go much into the definition of the extensively studied term, and I won't be able to explain it in just a few words. In short, this is how I interpret it based on what I have read on the subject, metaphysically and spiritually speaking, and I am by no means an expert, but I will try to do my best.

You come to the world, and your soul is pure light, ready to inhabit your body and live a human experience that lasts for a certain amount of time on earth. As time passes by, you build a personality to help you fulfill that human experience. The Ego uses some aspects of your skills in this physical life for you to create a false concept of yourself, an idea you end up believing and trusting. A set of "false beliefs."

Anxiety is one of the things that my Ego has formed in my life, and I was so used to it that I came to believe that anxiety is who I was. In reality, you are pure light. But your Ego has tried so hard to put particles in that light to make you believe you are a person you are not. The Ego is like a lousy screenwriter/director for your movie. You get so used to playing the part your Ego tells you to play that you become comfortable with it. But it's just an act. That is not who you are. The beautiful part is that you can fire your Ego at any moment and start discovering who you are, take control to direct, write and star in your own movie, which can be as brilliant as you can imagine it to be.

I didn't come up with this overnight; I had to dig deep for a while, and I am still in a constant path of self-discovery and evolution. In other words, I still have fights with my Ego. It is no longer the screenwriter/director of my movie, but sometimes it ends up doing unwanted special effects. It is the one that manages to put the anxiety monster on the scene from time to time. Continually, I have to use methods and tools to remember who I am.

When I started to play with these notions, I discovered several things about the role that my Ego wanted me to play. And it was painful but necessary. I had engraved a list of insecurities and a feeling of unworthiness that I was unable to explain, until I realized that I needed to let things go. Forgive and forget. For many years my Ego told me I was so unworthy, and it happened quietly. When I was a child, I believed that I was terrible with numbers and that I was always going to be, and because someone told me back then that people that were awful with math were bad in life, I believed that I was doomed to be unsuccessful. When I was a teen, I thought that I was ugly because some boys in high school decided to rate the girls in the class, putting me at the bottom of the list. When I was in college, I thought I was less than the rest of my friends because I was not in a stable relationship or couldn't even find a date.

The list goes on. Fortunately, for us humans, there is always another side that helps us to stay above this. Again, I will allow you to call it the name you want, but for me, that other part is something inside you, the part that counters the Ego. I am talking about the "Spirit," also known as the voice of your heart. The real you. No matter what happens in your life, you have deep dreams, things that make you "the real you," the things that make you happy. Sometimes we feel it, and sometimes we don't. Usually, anxiety crushes that voice. But, equally, as the Ego puts that set of false beliefs, your spirit works on countering them with "real ones," even if you are aware of this or not. The problem is that anxiety clouds you and doesn't let you understand what your spirit is trying to tell you. The magic formula to take that cloud away is to LET THINGS GO.

I needed to be able to re-discover who I was and let go of the past. Therapy was not doing that for me completely, and because I felt something was missing I searched for an alternative. I will tell you my story, and you can take it with a grain of salt if you want to, but it worked for me, and it might work for you. Ultimately is your choice, but I am guessing, if you are reading this book it is because you are open to finding new methods and tactics. I was desperate to reconnect with my soul. You can call it coincidence, and I will call it synchronicity. It is something that you have in your life, like the way the universe shows you the right path through the people around you and your experiences in the right perfect moment. So, a friend of mine introduced me to Carolina, a medium that works sort of like a translator between you and your spirit guides. Since I was already a believer that there is spiritual guidance both in the physical and non-physical world, I gave it a try. Carolina was the person that introduced me to a different concept of the Ego and has helped me to interpret situations and emotions through a spiritual path. Since the very first telephone conversation with her, I started experiencing a connection with that guidance. She explained to me that those guides are not in the business of foretelling your future. They want to help you to understand why you are living the experiences that you are living, and provide you tools to help you achieve your purpose in this human life. Through mediums like her, they show examples and give you messages that you can understand and use in your current situations and challenges to improve your life and fulfill your purpose. In a year of working along with her, doing exercises, and reinterpreting my life experiences, I was able to overcome more fears and discover myself in more ways than all the years of therapy for anxiety that I have experienced. I don't want to diminish the work and the great benefits of other kinds of treatment. As you may already know, I think you need to use all the methods you can, and therapy helped me also to be open to discuss my feelings and identify my triggers. But the spiritual guidance I found with Carolina is overall what has worked best for me. This approach switched my mindset. It helped me to understand that whatever I want to achieve or overcome needs a profound work from my part, but that I have the power in me to do so. Also, that I was never and will never be alone in the process. The reason why I think none of the other methods worked permanently before was simple: **no therapy, pill, medium, method will work if you are not willing to work on yourself and commit to feeling good.** You have to make a commitment to discover who you really are, drop the act, even if this means that you need to feel and change certain things on the road. And then, you have to honor that discovery.

There was one exercise that helped me, particularly with the letting go part. I made a list of all those things that my Ego had made me believe; a list of Ego traits, of all those particles that were clogging my light since I was a little child. I had to remember situations, experiences with a lot of people, and identify not only all of what was clouding my wellbeing but a whole lot of emotions different than anger and sadness that I was nurturing inside my soul. The deep-digging was one of the most painful exercises I ever had to do. But thanks to that exercise, I was able to finally see the awful role that my Ego had set me to play in my movie. My constant need to be recognized, accepted, and a weird addiction I developed for approval, that was holding me back and charging my monster, was all a con-job from my Ego.

Then, I had to read out loud one by one the points in that list and commit myself to let them go, thus taking away their power over me. In the end, it was like "Marie Kondo-ing" myself. I was getting rid of the things that were not allowing me to be happy. The list was bigger than I thought, but amazingly it was like throwing tons of bags filled with garbage. Once I finished, I prayed to fill that now empty space with my light. A light that actually was always there, but my Ego didn't let me see. I cried for a while, I burned the paper, and that was it. I was light as a feather.

What happened in the months after the experience was somehow surprising. At first, I was going through life like a phoenix, and I felt triumphant, empowered, like *Captain Marvel,* after absorbing the photon energy. Soon I discovered I had angered the Ego and that it was determined to take away my new superpowers. So, it sent the anxiety monster to attack back, and unexpectedly, fight full force. It was so mad that it summoned all my fears and my phobias as well. It was not letting me get rid of those particles that quickly. Little did it know, this time was different.

What the exercise gave me were the tools I needed to let things go before they put an imprint on me or before I engage with extreme, impulsive, and adverse reactions —the capacity to move on without overthinking on a problem or situation. I was now identifying those things that bothered me so easily and was able to recognize and embrace my emotions. I was aware of my ability to put my stuff on hold, rethink, and continue as needed. I stopped also trying to control all the outcomes, realizing that sometimes things are beyond our control. Most importantly, I started to see my anxiety monster triggers crystal clear. Such clarity helped me to learn to let things go, and my life changed. Sometimes it is more difficult to do than others, but I guess it is all about practice and getting better. And trust me, the universe will keep sending you situations and people for you to practice with until you learn your lesson. Have you ever questioned, "why this always has to happen to me?" Here's why; the universe sent you a test and you refuse to learn from it. So similar situations keep repeating in your life and you need to work hard not for the test itself, but to identify and apply the lesson behind. Once you learn it, you move on. You let it go. If you don't, you are calling a new test on the same subject. Like back in school, when you found yourself failing a class, the only way to pass is with practice and a lesson learned.

If I feel that something is bothering me, or that I have an unresolved situation and I can't let go, I write it down. I also write my desire to want this situation to be resolved but not saying how, because I don't want to focus on the outcome, which is out of my control. I trust that the universe will put everything into place for me to learn the lesson and find a resolution, in perfect synchronicity and timing, and then I let it go. I have faith that whatever happens in each case is what's best for my journey. I forgive the feeling, the person (if involved), and myself. I say a prayer, burn the paper, and see it disappear in front of my eyes. As it burns and visually disappearing, I am, in a way more understandable to my logic, letting it go.

I have to ask the following questions when something is not working: Is there something I can do? Is there a solution I can find right now? These questions help me to take action if needed.

The tricky part is the "forget." When I say forget, I am not talking about ignoring the situation or person. I forget about the negative feeling. I imagine a light taking its place. Just with that act of faith, I have many times encountered inspiration, or I was prone to an action that led me to resolve a situation or to stop thinking and obsessing about things. Sometimes the solutions are presented in an opportunity, something I read, even a song I hear that inspires me to do something else that helps me move on or also just put an end to that chapter of life. In times when you don't know what to do just close your eyes and imagine that light entering you. Ask for the negative feeling to be removed by that light. Believe that it can help you to find a solution. This exercise is basically calling your guides and ask them for help and most likely they will send the inspiration, the idea, the person you need. It is as simple as that.

If I feel I have things left unsaid to a person I speak and ask before I let assumptions consume me. The anxiety monster loves assumptions, so I don't even let it go there. I ask the person directly, and if for any reason I can't, I try to write them a letter. I express in writing how I feel, I am direct, and say all that I need to tear the walls down. In terms of conflict with another person, you have to know that there are always two sides. You have to give the other person a chance to explain his or her hand. Sometimes the conflict remains unresolved, sometimes the other person doesn't even reply to you, and that is okay. Just knowing you did your best and took the lead on trying to resolve a conflict helps. Please remember, you are not responsible for other people's happiness; you only have to seek yours. So now the battle is on their side, and there is nothing you can do about it. Could you put it on paper, burn it and let it go?

I encourage you to try to think about the things that bother you, the recurrent problems you find, and the challenges that anxiety has placed on you. I encourage you to believe that those negative things and false beliefs are not who you are. Think about your dreams, the things that inspire you, the things you like, the things you enjoy. What motivates you? Do you have a dream unfulfilled? How can you bring it back into your life and make it a reality? I invite you to discover your spirit, your inner voice, the voice of your heart, in any way possible. You have nothing to lose. Just like you, I have been trying method after method, and I found them all interesting and useful, but I got to tell you, reconnecting to your true self and your spirit will allow you to liberate yourself from those things that no longer bring you joy. The access to your true self is like having your own inner Marie Condo organizing you inner-soul cabinets. Or if you think there is something else that can help you to achieve this, try it! All that matters is that you find your true self, let the light through, and keep directing, writing, and staring in your movie. And yes, if you ask me, singing like Elsa from the top of your lungs from time to time also helps.

LESSON: Letting things go is an art that requires you to start a path of self-discovery, where you will be able to get the tools necessary to stop getting imprinted with negative emotions and false connotations of yourself. It requires practice and patience but will provide you with unlimited freedom and wellbeing.

TIPS:

- Making the list of Ego traits is a very personal exercise. If you want to try it, make it when you are alone and not bothered by anyone. You will need a few hours. Think of situations and people in your life that have made you feel a negative emotion, but don't put the blame on them. Think about how you felt and write it down. You can make it as extensive as you want, and go as far in your past as you want. Burning the paper has more than a metaphorical significance. You might encounter yourself writing things that no one else should see. If you feel vulnerable doing this exercise, don't force it. You will be able to do it on your terms if this is something you want to try. Also, please keep it safe! Don't burn your house! Put the paper on your kitchen sink, or outside on a fire pit, burn it where is safe, or if you don't like fire use a paper shredder.
- Instead of a list of past Ego traits, you can start with more recent situations. The exercise is the same and is also personal.
- Believe in the power of your light and the power from the universe to help you let things go and find inspiration.
- Forgive the situation or person with whom you are having difficulties. Then forget the emotion and be ready to move on.

MAY YOUR LOVE AND COMPASSION BE STRONGER THAN YOUR FEARS

"Fear is the path to the dark side. Fear leads to anger. Anger leads to hate. Hate leads to suffering."

—Yoda, Star Wars

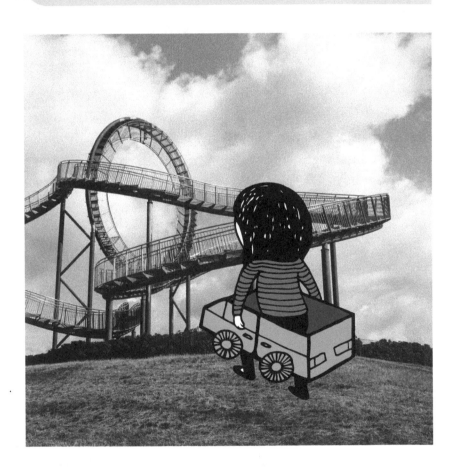

f anxiety had a best friend, it would be fear. And no, it wouldn't look like the cute character in *Inside Out*. Fear is as ugly and as dark as it gets. It can consume you silently if you let it. However, fear is not necessarily a bad sign, most of the time. As I mentioned in a previous chapter, fear can be the invitation of the universe for you to try something new, to learn, or to change something. It can put you on alert and awake your senses. And to act on that feeling is your decision to make. What you decide to do with fear can make all the difference in the world. It can also paralyze you, preventing you from learning and grow. And the inability to act can make you fall in anger or despair. Fear is fuel. It all depends on which side of the road you want to pursue.

What I am about to say to you might sound like a cliché, but I can assure you it's not. You can turn that fear fuel into love and compassion to start seeing life from a different perspective and heal everything you need. And when I say everything, I mean EVERYTHING. However, to allow that to happen, you need to be aligned. Alignment is a sense of inner wellbeing or connection with your soul (or spirit if you prefer to name it that way.) In other words, it is when you can release your fears easily and get tuned with your true self, who you are: your pure essence of light and love. When you are aligned, you feel good, when you are not, you feel bad. It's that simple. That is the compass you need to understand alignment. And it is okay that you not always tuned in and is natural to feel fear. However, you need to know that when you don't feel right, when you are not aligned, that's when fear stays in command. The important thing is that you can always find ways to realign.

Here's a story that might seem banal, but it taught me a great lesson about fear and love, and helped me understand how everyone has that aligning power. It all started with my fear of roller coasters. I used to be one of those persons that you see on the line with a terrified face instead of an excited one. My husband loves all those things; he enjoys extreme experiences and sports. Before I had kids, a few times, I went with him to theme parks, and I was very reserved with roller coasters. Despite his efforts, there were certain ones that I refused to get on. Fast forward to having two kids and moving to Florida. Theme parks are our thing now. It is an easy, two-hour drive from home, and there you have an utterly fantastic getaway. With them, I started to try to enjoy and see these parks with different light.

Still, the roller coasters seemed scary, having the anxiety monster terrifying me even more. I can't tell you the number of times that I had to get out of a long line because I was getting a panic attack from a roller coaster. However, life always has a way to test our limits and dare us. Because YOU HAVE TO LEARN THE LESSON, I think that is why God sent me Eva, my oldest one. My daughter started growing up and it was like the universe was telling me, "so do you think you can control things or control someone, uh? Go ahead, try with this one and let me know how it goes." She is one of those fearless, free-spirited, strong-willed children. These are somehow extraordinary traits to have, but as a mother with anxiety, I knew this was going to be a challenge. She loves roller coasters and enjoys anything that entails having some adrenaline rush. She even did parasailing when she was eight years old!

She pushes me to try new things and to take risks, and she does it with love. She has taught me to challenge my fears and discover my bravery, inviting me to see the world through her eyes. She was determined to stop my fear of roller coasters. So, inspired by her, I went in ones that, in past years, I did not dare to try. Believe it or not, she re-trained me, and I started to enjoy them! More than that, I was so glad that I could finally share these experiences with her. The happiness on her face is everything to me! Still, there was one that was always a NO-NO for me. The Hollywood Rip Ride Rockit at Universal Studios. I was not able to do that one with her. I was somehow terrified! She always had her way of convincing me to do things. This time she asked: "Aren't you writing a book about fighting your fears?" I was left speechless. She was right! How could I tell others to stop having fears when I was not able to face mine? Then she played an even bigger card. "Also, you always say moms do whatever for their kids. Do this for me, mama. Pleaseeeee!" How could I say no! She took my hand, and we went there together. She saw how terrified I was, but she held my hand and even reminded me of my breathing exercises. She told me that there was a song I could play since she had ridden it before and already knew every detail about it. "Mama, you can put 'I will survive'." My legs were shaking once I sat down next to her, and she was laughing. "First, I was afraid, I was petrified..." and then as Gloria Gaynor kept singing, I lived one of the most amazing experiences ever! I conquered my fear, me! An anxious mom! A person that left the line so many times before. But I realized that I did it thanks to love. Inspired by my daughter's bravery, and her persuasive loving guidance, I released control, I surrendered. I faced my fear and understood that all you have to do is give yourself a chance to prove to yourself (not to anybody else) how strong you are.

Love is a strange force. When I think of the definition of it, I remember the movie *Interstellar*. Bear with me, once again. There is a scene where Dr. Brand (Anne Hathaway) explains it like this: "**Love** is the one thing we're capable of perceiving... that transcends dimensions of time and space. Maybe we should trust that, even if we can't understand it yet." We feel moved by the people we love as I felt with my daughter after convincing me to live the experience with her. When we are inspired by love we simply don't question it maybe because it is a force that we just don't understand but we have to trust. My daughter was so proud of me and proud of herself for finally convincing me to do one of her favorite things together. When we let fear get in the way, it prevents us from living amazing experiences with the people we love, particularly with our kids. They are little just once. If you think about it, we have them under our roof for such a small period of their lives. At that moment, I realized I was letting my fear not only taking opportunities away from me but also from my kids. "The things we do for love..." I thought and laughed.

I was thinking about how our children's love is a constant fuel. Erik, my youngest one, who is somehow different than my daughter, reserved just like me, and not that fearless, is the one that has shown me how I could feel deserving of unconditional love. After many decades of fearing rejection, feeling a need to be accepted, he brought my life a constant self-esteem boost, a little man that kisses me and looks at me like there is no one else in the world comparable to me. Thanks to both of them and the way I love them and the way they love me, I have been discovering that this is the force that I need to use to surpass anything, to realign when I need to, and that sometimes I need their hugs and kisses more than they need mine. I wonder, if they love me that much, how come I continuously find myself not loving me as I should?

Yes, I know I don't have to explain love to you. You are a mom, so you know what I mean. You know what unconditional love is and what you are capable of doing for that love. You know that there is nothing impossible when you are powered by it, there is nothing you couldn't do. But despite this, you are still covered with fears. Why? I think the answer is straightforward: moms forget about loving themselves. We forget. We have everyone else in mind, but we are the last person on our list (if we even make it to the list,) and this has to change. We need to learn to love ourselves first because the lack of self-love is what opens the door to more fears.

Before becoming a mom, I thought I knew love. And in a way, I did. But it was very different. You never forget that day and how motherhood shifts you. It's like someone suddenly turns on a switch in your soul. Something that was dormant for years and then is lighting your entire world and giving you a different purpose. How you become a mom, it is irrelevant. What kind of mother you become it is irrelevant. We all endure an extraordinary transformation with the process, physically, mentally, and emotionally. Motherhood also brings other discoveries. For example, that indeed, you become a sort of life tour guide for some tiny humans that are now your responsibility; they learn and nurture from you. But in reality, they are your most prominent teachers, especially when it comes to face your fears. Because oh yes, motherhood brings you big worries, and the anxiety monster knows this.

You already have a set of fears and individual insecurities and then comes motherhood bringing brand new ones not only toward your new role but also, toward the safety of these creatures that you feel are yours to protect —an instant discovery. Since the moment I was pregnant I felt the need to protect them. As mothers, we are usually contemplating them, marveling in their development, but also terrified that someone or something can harm them. Anxiety increments that fear to levels that can spin your life out of control. When you let that fear drive your life, you can miss crucial moments in the life of your children, or prevent them from experiences they can enjoy just because of your anxiety.

You are not fully present. In other words, you are not enjoying that unconditional love; you are putting conditions to it instead.

When my anxiety was horrible a few years ago, I started to fear death. Fears of dying are natural in mothers, but we don't talk about this. You think about what can happen to them in case you are gone. Or even worse, about something happening to them. I think for a mother, there is no bigger fear than the fear of losing her kids.

This next topic can trigger some readers, so I am giving you heads up before we talk about losing a child. I saw my best friend going through this pain, and also how she was able to continue living and loving thanks to her other two children. But even having someone close to me enduring this experience, I think I didn't understand the feelings she went through. And because I didn't, I might have hurt her with my judgments and my response to my fears. I wish I could go back in time and be there for her in a more meaningful way because I wasn't and I regret that. After years I finally could see that a person's path to healing is personal and develops in her terms and timeline. The lesson I got from her was that the only way a person can keep pushing through after something like that is love. My friend, who I adore, has shown me how a mother who loses her child will never be the same; sometimes she cries, sometimes life gets hard when she remembers what happened, but love keeps her pushing through, and love still shines through despite it all. And experience makes her smile again and love life even more. She showed me that love is a healing power.

When you have someone close to you going through something like this you put things into perspective. We live in a chaotic world where we have news and social media every day, bombarding us with terrifying stories, and people are going through painful experiences and grief. We are dealing with having our kids participate in lockdown drills at school, and we endured challenging years like 2020 where the global pandemic turned everything upside down. So how can you not feel dragged into fears in such an environment? And, then the fear of losing something or someone we love kicks in and can make it challenging to handle when you have anxiety. Those fears disconnect you from your purpose, and with who you are.

For a while, I became obsessive, paranoiac, and even a little bit hypochondriac. The more I was thinking about death my anxiety started to become stronger. I became fixated with the stories I read on social media or watched on the news, and I was again overthinking about the future, with the constant "what would happen if..." thought. That made me extremely reserved. I was avoiding risks, scared of trying new things, and seeing danger everywhere. Also, I stopped doing the things that I used to enjoy, and without noticing, I was becoming a very controlling and fearful mother.

Then came this realization. That fear of losing something or someone you love is preventing you from living and enjoying the time you have now with those who you love or the experience that you love. That fear makes you focus on the problems and the threats instead of allowing yourself to lose control and just get carried away by love. We don't know how long we will be on this earth. The bottom line is that we are here now, sharing life and love with our families and friends, so we need to enjoy every single second while we still can, no matter the experience or the challenge we are facing.

I took matters into my own hands and focused on identifying the things that were affecting my wellbeing the most. I restricted the way I consumed social media and the news, mainly when it's about traumatic stories. I don't let the negative narrative drag me. I don't watch the news that much anymore. I found other ways of being informed and learned to take precautions when needed. Social media was also a trigger, so I started to unfollow people and pages that were just too toxic for me.

I understood that all I need to do is feel love and gratitude for my own life, my family, my own experiences (even the bad ones,) and then enjoy every single second that life gives me with the people I love. Love and appreciation make me feel good, no matter what I am facing, and then I feel aligned. Also, there is a significant factor for compassion. People suffer, and the best way to help others is not getting involved in their experiences and choices but offering them our love and understanding. We need to be able to love and heal ourselves first to offer that kind of help if someone asks for it. I wrote this book as part of my healing process and as my words were coming from a place of love, I could use the declarations and my stories cathartically. Slowly I discovered that my words were inspiring others but I don't want to impose my philosophies. My journey and my lessons are ultimately mine but if my story inspires you and speaks to you I am honored. If I learned a lot on my journey, why not share my experiences with others? Most of the time, help comes in the works of inspiration, not by forcing change on others. My only intention with what you are reading is to inspire you. You can take what you want and release what you think is not for you. I will not feel offended and we can still be friends.

The relationship and the love I share with my kids has been a prominent and fundamental motor in my way to recovering. Eventually and ultimately, they are going to have lives of their own outside my roof, and there is nothing I can do, even if I want to, I will not be able to control them. Never. Because let's be honest, we do want to be able to manage them. We want to put them in a bubble and make them so safe they don't have to feel pain ever. But this is impossible. They have to live, and make mistakes, know heartache and deception; deal with their own fears, and overcome all of that just the way we did. And the only way to understand this and letting go is trough love. As mothers, we do all we can to make them feel loved. And you know when they get sick, or when they cry, they find comfort in our arms and our love helps them to heal. Why can't we use love to improve ourselves?

They need to have me in my best, so I have to love me first. I started to love the person I am now, not the one I was or the one that I want to become. I began to work in the person I am and soon started seeing how I was making better decisions. I had better results, was manifesting great things into my life, doing the things that I never thought I was going to be able to do, and fulfilling my dreams. The best part is that I love myself more than ever.

What you need to understand is that you need to choose how to act on fear. You can remain frozen by it or you can let love inspire you and turn it into proactive fuel. When we have a problem, face an awkward situation, try to make an important decision, or when we think of losing our health, our loved ones, our money, our jobs, we need to be guided by love and not by fear. The compass is there; you are the only one that can choose which direction to take. Fear won't lead you to a solution or a positive change or thought. Love does, always. Loving our bodies, our minds, our life, despite any setbacks or difficult situations, is the only way that we can enjoy our time here. Loving your children, your spouse, your friends, your family, instead of thinking that somehow you will lose them, will inspire you to enjoy time with them as much as you can. You might be missing great opportunities just by being paralyzed by fear. I am not implying that you won't feel fear anymore. Of course, you will! and you must! What matters is that you can quickly recognize fear as a signal that you need to let love in and let it guide you. When you take action from a place of love, it will direct you exactly where you need to be. It will get you further away if you do it from a space of fear.

In the end, every day is a roller coaster. I encourage you to start each day by knowing that you have the love inside you, and the love of others to support you. You can go up or down, take twists and turns, even feeling that you are going backward. But each day is an exhilarating ride you need to learn to enjoy. Let love take control of you, and you will see you have nothing to fear. Now conquer your Everest, ride your Rip Ride Rockit whatever it may be, as many times you need. You will see that when you do it you will want to repeat the ride, and again, and again. You will survive.

 LESSON: You already know the power of love. Use it as your most significant shield against anxiety. Let love replace every fearful thought, particularly when you think about yourself, and take action from a place of love.

 TIPS:
- Try to see the world through your children's eyes, and you will find powerful discoveries.
- Put yourself as a priority. Love the person you are now. Don't think about the one you were or the one you want to become.
- Don't let the experiences of others enhance your fears. Treat the stories of others with compassion and love but with the understanding that they are not your experiences.

- Know that your kids are individuals that have to learn but also need you in your best.
- Try to be inspiring instead of controlling. Remember, you can't change others, you can only motivate them through love.

DON'T GIVE IN TO JUDGMENTS

"Never forget what you are. The rest of the world will not.
Wear it like armor, and it can never be used to hurt you."

—Tyrion Lannister, *Game of Thrones*

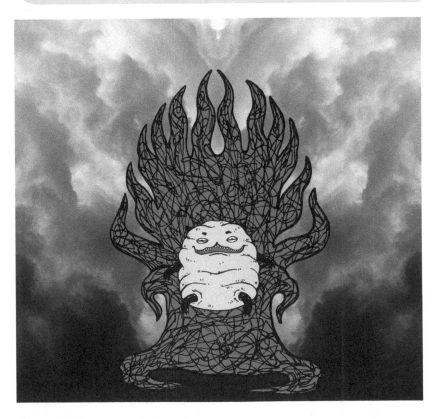

One thing you need to know about me is that I love *Game of Thrones*. Scratch that. I am obsessed with *Game of Thrones*, the series. Yes, even with "that" ending. Aside from its mythology and fantasy components, the story fascinated me for the complexity of its conflicts. For years fans like me were glued to the TV wondering who would end up sitting on the throne. Spoiler alert ahead (although at this point if you don't know this I am assuming you don't care about it); there was no throne for anybody, there was a melted one. Yes, no one got it (and I am not talking about Arya Stark,) and the most unthinkable group of people ended up ruling Westeros. Now let's get to my point. One day while I was watching an episode, somehow, I ended up comparing the conflicts from G.R.R. Martin's fiction to the mom wars. Because let me tell you something, mom wars are real! Let's call it "Game of Moms."

When you play the game of moms, "you win, or you die." Okay, you won't die, but you can get extremely anxious. Of course, we are not that brutal and fortunately, we don't have dragons, wildfire, or use other dangerous weapons in such wars. But believe me, we can find similar components of betrayal, backstabbing, hypocrisy, and ruthless picking and judgment between "mom houses." And all for nothing.

In the battle for the throne, meaning for "which kind of mom does it better," in the end, no one will sit on it just like in the show. We can think we are like *Cersei* or *Daenerys*, but in reality, all moms, regardless of which kind, are more like a version of *Jon Snow*. WE KNOW NOTHING. All of us are learning, all of us struggle, and all of us have a difficult time one way or the other. We do our best we can because motherhood is not easy. Not even for Kate Middleton. However, we end up tearing each other apart using the most dangerous of weapons: judgments. Mom wars had given me so much unnecessary anxiety that I realized I had to avoid them at all costs.

The house of the Stay at Home Moms (AKA SAHM) and the house of Working Moms are the strongest and biggest ones. Imagine each one claiming they have it worse than the other hence, they are better moms because they had to work harder and have more significant challenges. In my only first decade of motherhood, I have seen enough of the battle between these houses, and to this day, I still don't understand the need to proclaim which group is better. The truth is, no one is. The problem of motherhood is that we don't see each other as sisters. We have created these ridiculous divisions trying to answer the question of "who can have it all?" and in the end, the competition generates frustration, anger, and anxiety.

Other subgroups have developed like the single moms (who by the way I personally think they are absolute heroes,) the divorce moms, the PTA moms, or the entrepreneurial moms. We also have the married once or more moms, the helicopter moms, the clueless moms, the teacher moms, the anti-vaxxer moms, the fit moms, and the list can go on and on and on...

Let's try to think about the question again. "Can we have it all?" For me is even stupid that we ask ourselves this because "all" is a different concept for everybody. The sooner you get that the better. However, somehow moms instead of helping each other, we end up competing in order to validate our choices. Whose kid is smarter the house cleaner or whose partner gives the best present on Valentine's Day? Who has better vacations? Which parenting style is best? Whose kid does more extracurricular activities? The best way to show others they are winning the game of moms is to display noticeable results on social media to get said validation. The perfect pictures and stories try to show the rest that they are, in fact, better, happier, and "have it all" figured out, perpetuating the model of "a mom has to be perfect, or she is not a good mom."

Battles take place in scenarios such as the playground, school recitals, groups of friends having drinks, and even family reunions. There is one ruthless place where you can see a dramatic display of conflict: The mom "insert category here" FB group. One single misfortunate comment in the wrong chat can turn you into *Catelyn Stark* attending a cybernetic version of a Red Wedding however instead of a wedding, it's just a FB post. And sometimes it has even worse consequences. The other day I read the story of a mom who turned to one of those groups to get advice about her son's flu, and some moms started giving her inaccurate medical information that ended up costing her son's life. And there came more judgments and more negativity.

The war was extremely evident when in the midst of the pandemic, parents were forced to decide how they were going to continue their children's education after months of quarantine. The decision was not easy for anybody, but the judgments were crystal clear out in the open. The situation repeats itself over and over in different circles, events, and circumstances. No matter what you decided to do there was always a mom or several out there judging others. How can we stop this madness? I got to say that not all groups or moms behave like this. But we need to find a way that we stop tearing each other apart because it happens even in our closest circles of friends and a lot of times unnoticeable.

You have to remember something. Moms don't use swords but words, which sometimes can be more harmful. It's like living in big fields cultivated by judgments. That's is why we hide our mental illness. We rather stay silent to avoid ending up without our heads for no reason, and we get consumed with doubts because of it. Judgments make us question our role and every single decision we make; thus, we end more confuse and fearful. And because we feel like failing, we feel worthless.

We are all judgmental somehow, it's in our nature. But I believe there is an awakening happening on how, by reducing the judgment, our wellbeing increases. The philosophy behind this is the following. When we throw judgments toward another human being, most likely, it's directed to oneself. The problem is that we don't know it. We believe we have the answers to other people's struggles; we think that we can fix them. In reality, there is something inside of us that makes us uncomfortable, and we mirror that feeling instead of trying to fix what is happening inside of us. And moms can be cruel in their judgments.

When I decided to stay at home after becoming a mom, I received all kinds of judgments from my friends and family. People don't do it intentionally most of the times, and usually, it starts with questions or small comments that initially seem harmless like "Oh, you have all the time in the world because you don't work" or, "how can you be so tired and look like that if you are at home all the time." It also happens with body language. When I tell other moms that I am a writer, sometimes I get what I call "the look," the one that immediately translates into "that is not a real job." Once a friend even asked me how we were able to travel living with just one income. Or another day, I forgot to put earrings and another friend was perplexed, like if I had forgotten to feed my children or something like that. And when it came to my anxiety, it was even worse. "It's all in your head." "OMG, you are so dramatic." "Don't pass your insecurities to your children."

The key is in the reaction to judgments and not playing the game. If we don't engage, it will pass. And that's the end of it. If you suddenly encounter yourself being the one giving the judgment, try to ask yourself what is bothering you, what do you need to fix in you. Judging others takes our energy away. But the worst part is that if we open the door to those judgments, we end up believing in them. So, the comment that starts innocently can become a belief, a self-judgment that our Ego turns into a false fact, and those are extremely dangerous. It happened to me. There were moments that I let those judgments affected me, and suddenly I was saying awful things to myself, like "I am worthless," "What I do has no value," or "I look miserable." Then I was in constant search for validation, but it was driving me crazy, and my anxiety got much worse. I was not only repeating those negative things, I believed they were my truth.

Until I decided to focus on me and accepting my flaws, I think I took the first step when I decided to be open about my anxiety. I wanted to get better, but also, I felt the need to show others that motherhood is not shinning stars and rainbows all the time, and I was refusing to participate in the ridiculous mom wars. Also, because I realized people usually judge anxiety without even knowing what it is, like people on planes without kids who look at you like you are a monster when your toddler has a tantrum. The same thing happens when it comes to mental health. People have no idea how to respond because even when all human beings deal with certain levels of anxiety, their experience is different. But if we educate, lift, and complement each other, we all can live better lives. Also, when we respect other people's decisions and choices, even when for us, they won't work, we should practice praising more often, and see the good in others. We can learn so much from each other, especially from other moms.

If you see a mom alone in the playground looking confused, approach her and talk. Or practice compassion and offer your help to the mom in the parking lot yelling at her child, this could be you. If another mom is sick and has no one to help her, go to her house and at least keep her company. You can also make her some tea. We are all on the same boat, figuring all this out. No mom is better than the other. We all have our talents and things that can be improved. We may have different approaches and have differences, but we share one thing that makes us equal, we are all mothers. Plus, not every mom has a village.

Don't get me wrong. Mom tribes can also be very positive. You can always have that group of moms that are different from each other, and you end up learning from them and them from you, creating a lovely bond that can last a lifetime. If you have such a tribe, you are fortunate. Cultivate those friendships because these are the ones that you need to maintain. Any relationship needs nurturing from both sides, so take care of those moms that are in your tribe as they take care of you. And try to stay away from judging as much as you can.

So if you get accidentally caught in the Game of Moms don't try to be a *Cersei* or *Daenerys*. Be a *Jon Snow*. You probably, in fact, may know nothing, but in terms of participating in a mom war, you can always say, "I don't want it."

 LESSON: When you receive a judgment, remember not to engage after it happens. Let it pass by. If you are passing judgment, reflect on what is bothering you inside and on what you need to work. The further you are from judgments, the closer you are to aligning with well-being.

 TIPS:
- Accept other moms as equal in the motherhood experience, despite what kind of mom you consider yourself to be.

- Practice gratitude and compassion. Offer your help to anther mom; it's the best feeling in the world.
- Avoid participating in groups and conversations where judgments are the main topic.
- If you judge, know that you can always examine yourself and fix inside of you what is bothering you.
- **In the name of all things holy: DO NOT ASK OR GIVE MEDICAL ADVICE ON FB GROUPS OR OTHER SORTS OF CHATS.**

BE AWARE THAT YOU DON'T NEED VALIDATION

"If everybody were like everybody else, how boring it would be.
The things that make me different are the things that make me, me!"

—Piglet, Winnie the Pooh

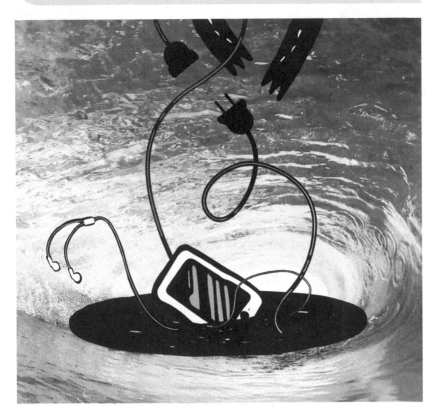

One day a friend called me to talk about her anxiety. I am glad that since I am entirely open talking about this, a lot of people have come forward and told me their stories. I am always happy to help if I can, and if they ask me, or at least I am willing to listen and be supportive. She had got her diagnosis recently, and we started talking about the steps she was taking for healing, and how the main trigger for her panic attacks and other symptoms were coming from her job. She was so proud that she was going to start therapy, but then she said, "I want them to take me seriously. I don't want them to think this is fake." This statement caught my attention because this is precisely a big problem for us while trying to recover. We get anxious about what other people think of us or how they will react when you decide to be open with your anxiety, assuming that they immediately will put a label on you simply because they don't understand what anxiety is. We constantly feel we need to justify our condition to feel validated because this is a hard thing to explain, mostly because it's an "invisible" condition.

If you break your leg and you need a cast to repair, nobody will question it. But when you have a mental illness, how can you convince others that you need specific treatment or procedures to heal? My question goes further, why do we need to? Why, on top of what we have to deal with our anxiety, we seek validation from others and justify ourselves? You don't need this. The less you try, the better you will feel. But I understand, this is not easy. It's probably one of the hardest things I had to overcome in my journey.

It's exhausting explaining to others why you need therapy, why you take pills, why you have to retreat from time to time, or why you act the way you do. Something started happening to me, and as I felt misunderstood, I started to feel like a victim. I started saying things like, "Others are attacking me" "The universe is against me" "Others are extremely unfair," or "Why me?." I was putting the blame elsewhere and doing nothing to change what I was going through. It made me justify the way I was feeling and the way people reacted, but all I was feeling was anger. The more victimized I felt, the more I was seeking for an external source for healing, like a magical cure to anxiety or expecting an expert miracle worker to tell me what to do. Also, I found myself in a constant pettish mood, and I started complaining about everything and everyone, nothing around me seemed to fit. I rarely had something positive to say, and I was in a permanent state of irritability.

I was feeling miserable, and falling into depression. While I was trying to get other people to "take me seriously" or looking for something external and magical to "fix me," I was also using my anxiety as an excuse to remain numb. The way to healing from a mental illness is confusing and very personal. It is even more difficult when you are constantly trying to validate your condition to others, because you are doing too many things at the same time, and the monster knows that well.

Again, sometimes the universe has weird ways of sending messages. Someone told me an analogy about how being a writer of different genres or having several books written is like being an air traffic controller, and I immediately applied it to anxiety. It's like trying to land many planes at once as your mind serves as the traffic controller, but you need to **concentrate your efforts into landing ONE plane first.** When it comes to anxiety or any mental illness, usually, what keeps us frozen is the battle inside our head —the colliding million thoughts, precisely like the traffic controller. For the anxious person, it seems like we need to put all the planes on land at the same time, or nothing will work. However, that plane you need to land first is your well-being. Your problems, other people's actions, your daily tasks, every single different plane will follow once you feel good because you will figure out everything else with ease. But if you are in a place of anger, anguish, despair, and victimization, you will overthink, even more, and that means having to deal with more planes on your radar.

In a moment, I was like this. Too overwhelmed with thoughts, too confused, too tired, and also anxious, with many ideas and planes for me to handle. My mind and life were juggling things like the unkempt house, the kids you need to look after, the relationship with your partner that needs nourishing. But wait, there's more: you're the body that has not bounced back, your career goals that have taken a step back, the shower you haven't had, or the expectations from others that you want to fulfill. It's exhausting and even more so when you are trying to keep your anxiety under control. You'll crash all your planes if you continue like this. It takes a simple decision to land the plane of wellbeing first, your choice for feeling good, whatever it means, and whatever it takes.

I was tired of being the victim, trying to seem perfect, and not getting anything solved. At that moment, I decided that I needed to be as public as I could about my anxiety. Until then, I was either hiding my condition or forcibly trying to expect others to understand it. Being silent or perpetuating a victim mentality can be easy, but by doing so, I was taking away my power to heal. Trust me, the power is in you, probably dormant, but you have all the possibility to awaken it. Until that happens, there is no pill, therapy, or any other anxiety remedy that will work. One thing I understood in the process and that I want to tell you is that you have to make the decision to work in your well-being. You need to understand that even though there are a lot of resources out there for help and guidance YOU are the one that has to do the work.

You have to decide to look into yourself and put your well-being as a priority; you have to choose to feel good, without seeking validation or victimizing yourself. You have to believe you are braver than you think. You have to commit to working on yourself without meeting the expectations of others and at your own pace.

A few years ago, I started to share my experiences through my blog that has now turned into the book you are reading. I decided I was not going to be embarrassed about anything anymore, and Momxious helped me explore my feelings by being as honest as possible while being able to share my truth. I not only felt liberated and empowered but, I believed I was contributing to the conversation about mental illness, especially among mothers that felt my message was relatable. The more I wrote, the more responses I got, and a tighter Momxious community was growing. Even people that I would have never guessed had similar experiences wrote me and felt encouraged to speak or look for help. You are not alone in this fight. You can start feeling better today, but it has to be YOUR choice.

We are not "anxiety," so don't let your mental illness define you. You can reinvent yourself as many times as you want. You are the sum of many ingredients that make you a unique and delicious recipe. Find the flavors, play with the elements, and learn to identify them. You can add new ones as you move forward. Being a mom is already hard, who are we kidding? No one has it easy, not even that well put-together lady you see every morning on time in the school carpool line, with the perfect hair and the spotless clean car.

I already told you how giving into judgments can blur your vision. The same thing happens with seeking validation or making assumptions. Instead of seeking validation, let's find support and encouragement. Instead of hiding, let's talk about our condition and educate others. Instead of feeling self-conscious, let's choose to feel good. Instead of complaining, let's practice gratitude, and instead of making assumptions, let's ask others directly and get a clear response from them when you need to.

Once you stop feeling like the universe is against you, you can think more clearly. By trying to solve everything at once, you would get more confused. You need to do whatever it takes to feel good and keep your anxiety monster at bay first. You need to think of loving yourself first, on being your best version, and then figure out the rest, step by step, including helping others if that is in your agenda. It's not being selfish; it's prioritizing your sanity. And a lot of our overthinking and planes flying around come from that need for validation. You don't have to hide who you are or what you feel because of others. What you need to do is own who you are and your decision to recover and start feeling good. Send those validations to the trash and remember to land your well-being plane first. After that, all the landings will be smooth, and your skies will open up.

 LESSON: Your need to convince others how you feel in order to get validation is taking away your power to heal. Choose to feel good regardless of what others may think, and you will find the right directions and mechanisms for your well-being. Think about educating others when talking about your anxiety instead of feeling like a victim.

 TIPS:
- Use your emotions like a thermostat. Aim to feel good most of the time, so when your feelings tell you that you are on the low side, you can take immediate action.

- Stop blaming others about your problems and your condition. Only you can change something inside you.
- Practice gratitude whenever you can.
- Don't try to fix everything at once.
- In your journal, create a list of things, and the reason why you love yourself and read them daily. I have a positive description about myself that I read as often as needed to remind me that I am valuable and I need self-love. You can do the same.

REMEMBER THAT MOTHERHOOD IS NOT A COMPETITION

"After a while, you learn to ignore the names people call you and just trust who you are."

—Shrek

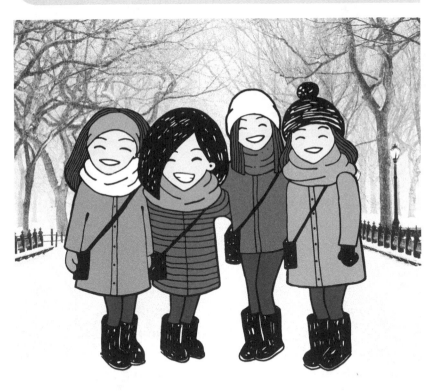

Now that I have talked about the mom wars and the validation we seek from others, we can talk about how to survive anxiety in a world where motherhood has become a competition. Motherhood is challenging, and no one speaks about it. Since the moment we get pregnant we feel the pressure, particularly from other moms, about how to handle your new role. We start receiving an immeasurable amount of unsolicited advice and the latest information about up and coming issues in "MommyVille." No matter how many parenting books you read, diapers you changed, or kids you babysat, nothing prepares you for motherhood. And your first child doesn't equip you for the second. But you get there, and all you hear is that you should not only be happy the entire time while listening to unwelcome tips on how to be a "good mother." No wonder we all feel like a failure at some point and get anxious and depressed for not meeting those expectations or developing specific feelings.

Let's take celebrities for a fun example. There are women like Kate Middleton; you know the type who barely gain weight and look stunning the entire time. The world has watched in awe every time the Duchess of Cambridge has gone into labor only to appear even more perfect a few hours later. She didn't even look like she just gave birth but more like she went to a dentist appointment instead and came out looking more glamorous than ever. And then you have celebs like Kim Kardashian or Jessica Simpson. Absolutely stunning women that no matter what, even when they are rich and famous and have access to all the chefs, massages, treatments, they gain so much weight and get so scrutinized and body shamed. We always compare ourselves to these women, and because we see how the world reacts to their pregnancies, we measure our levels to the same standards even when we are not famous; we shouldn't do that.

I am sure of something. Even the perfect Kate suffered some "pregnancy surprise," because yes, we all had those. From hemorrhoids to hyperemesis gravidarum. Maybe your feet got bigger, or you developed a curly section on your hair that not even the most potent keratin treatment can contain (true story!) I have heard all sorts of weird consequences from pregnancy. The truth is that all mothers suffered a transformation, and we should not compare to one another in such a negative way. Maybe we should just praise each other on the fact that no matter what each one of us, we did a great job! We did what we had to do to keep those little human beings safe in our bellies. And that's hard. Or even if you didn't go through that process yourself, you did the best you could! The process of becoming a mother regardless of the route is hard. Period.

Then we had to deal with the delivery. And I have just one thing to say here. This process is so unique for each woman that we should STOP, in the name of all the things holy, giving advice about this one to other women, unless you are her obstetrician. We get terrified for months because other moms have their own "Tales from the crypt, the delivery version." It's always someone that knows someone whose delivery was (insert traumatic experience.) Why people have to do that? I have no idea. If you are pregnant and reading this book, I can assure you, you will be fine, and you will do whatever it takes and the best you can do at that moment despite your friend's tale from the crypt. Avoid those conversations, or tell the person to stop.

Then we have the feeding battle. To breastfeed or not to breastfeed, that is the question. Some of us can do it some of us can't. AND THAT IS FINE!!! Feeding a kid, in general, is difficult, from the moment they are born. What is important is that you feed them the way you choose and the way you can, and this is no one else's business. You nurture your child, keep him alive and healthy, knowing that **your way** is the best.

And when you finally have that little creature in your arms, experiencing all sorts of feelings, and you are still clueless, but you are doing your best, the mom race begins. Scratch that, this starts even before: "Put makeup before your delivery. You need to look perfect for the picture." "How many gallons of milk you produce? I can barely keep all my milk production on the freezer!" "Aren't you going back to work?" "How can you get back to work so soon?" "What? Your kid doesn't speak (walk/potty trained/sleep all night/sleep alone/go to daycare/read/does algebra and astrophysics) already?" "So, how many extracurricular activities does your kid have?" "Are you telling me he doesn't have a schedule?"

Yes, I am going to stop right there, because there are tiny examples of the mom competition, extremely connected to the mom wars that I mentioned previously. The worst part is that we are extremely passive-aggressive and that's how moms hurt each other. It isn't enough to have to be a perfect mother, but also we need to raise perfect kids: the smartest, cleanest, well behaved, gifted, and talented children. Of course, we are going to develop some anxiety! And some more than others. Even sometimes accompanied by depression and other mental illnesses. What are we doing this to ourselves and other moms? There is no trophy at the end of the road, and it doesn't matter if you had a C-section or not, or how you feed your child, or if little Erik eats chicken nuggets instead of broccoli, kale, and protein! The only and most essential reward that a mom has at the end of the day is the smile in those little faces. That's all you need.

I gained 62 pounds with my second kid, and after almost seven years since he was born, I am not even close to my pre-kids size and weight. I have a child who for quite a while only ate meatballs, pizza, and grapes, and started talking after turning three. My daughter doesn't wear pink or like to dress up. They are not in a different activity each day of the week, and they misbehave regularly. Sometimes we just spend an entire weekend at home while skipping the shower routine, or I just put a Costco pizza in the oven because I can't deal with cooking. In the first years of motherhood, I was so anxious mostly because I felt like I was failing as a mother, thinking I was not good enough, and I was not making a sufficient effort. Little by little, I started owning my choices and not giving importance to the expectations of other moms and society of what a good mom is supposed to be. **A good mom is the one that is doing her best.** There is no award show for the mom of the year, no red carpet event for the best in the motherhood business, or great cash prizes. What matters is that you provide, within your capabilities, the best environment for your children. You do your best to have happy and healthy children, help them discover their strengths, not forcing them to become a better version of you, but helping them to become a better version of themselves through the years.

I got to say, all of this has escalated to epic proportions thanks to social media. If anxiety is a monster, social media is its favorite candy. The false representation of motherhood that is displayed online is overwhelming. I know it isn't easy, but you need to stop the urge to compare to others based on their social media platforms, which purpose is to appeal and sell an X factor. No mom is going to post their mess regularly. Some do it, and I love that! But almost no one would post about the ugly side of motherhood because it is considered parenthood heresy! A method I started using and has worked wonders for me is a daily detox from devices! Put your electronic devices down for an entire hour every day and regularly increase until you hit a 2-hour mark.

The problem is we get trapped, mostly with our phones, and then complain about not having time for other things. We also start developing an unhealthy relationship with others because of the illusion that these platforms provide.

You can try one hour in the morning and one in the evening. Use this time for yourself or to be with your family, where the real connection is needed. Also, while scanning your social media accounts, try to choose love instead of other negative emotion and abstain from comparisons. Try to celebrate what other people post, know that there is no perfection, and we are all struggling, learning, thriving, discovering. It's always lovely to see the successes of others or just the things that make them happy. Their life is not your life, and that's okay. Nobody knows what others are going through.

If you still want it to see it as a competition, then try this. Motherhood is a marathon where it's not important how fast you run it, or how well you trained —what you need to understand is that in this race there are no winners, no medals, and you need to pace yourself from time to time. It gives you courage when others cheer for you on the road, so do the same for them. If you see a fellow runner in need, assist them! And guess what? This marathon will never end, so don't rush it. Let's try to support each other and stop running; sometimes, is better to stop and look at the scenery. We are all doing just fine. Be proud of whatever you achieve daily, even if this is giving them or yourself a shower.

Remember you already hit the big prize and they call you mamma (or mommy, or mom, or mami, or mooooooooom!)

LESSON: Motherhood is not a competition. We are all doing the best we can, and all that matters is that you feel comfortable with your decisions and be unapologetic about them.

TIPS:

- When people give you unsolicited advice, try to listen to them. Don't take it personally. Decide if there's a piece of information you want to keep and disregard the rest. If this bothers you, tell them to stop, plain and simple.
- Abstain of comparisons. Especially when you are scanning social media accounts.
- Detox from your devices daily.
- Celebrate other people's achievements and milestones. You don't have to be in the same place they are because THEY ARE NOT YOU.
- Focus on your wellbeing and your children's happiness.

TAKE CARE OF YOURSELF, BE AWARE OF YOUR NEEDS

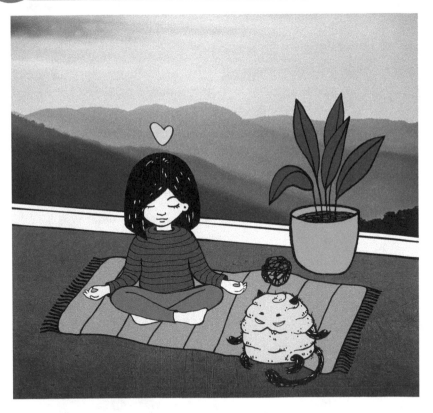

f there is a sin that moms commit is forgetting about themselves. We are natural nurtures who are always thinking about others. But what about us? What about our needs or dreams? We need to sacrifice many things while being mothers; there is no question about it, and please let's don't deny it. Especially when our kids are so little, and they depend on us to survive. However, as moms, we need to remember that if we are not happy, if we are not well, things won't run how they're supposed to in our families. Some people tend to say that moms are the heart of the family and others, that we are the brain. I am pretty sure we are the blood. We carry the oxygen and nutrients to our family organism. Life flows because of us. We are the ones that take care of any type of infection, and every single organ depends on us to function correctly. And what happens when the blood has a disorder? It needs treatment. I make this analogy to show you how important you are as a mom. If you ever feel underestimated, invisible, useless, incapable, mistreated, overwhelmed, pressured, remember you are the blood. You are vital, essential, exclusive, and no one else can do what you do.

Before becoming a mom and a writer I had different priorities and dreams. When I graduated from high school, I saw journalism as a suitable choice as opposed to dedicating my life to writing books. Back then, I wasn't even considering leaving my country, but things started to change, and a feeling of not belonging anywhere began to grow inside of me. After I graduated from college, a chain reaction of circumstances and opportunities led me to decide to leave Colombia. I came to the United States in 2002 and started my career as a journalist. I even had the chance to own my own magazine. I earned a Master's degree and was on the right path of meeting the expectations I had set for myself when I was younger. I already had my anxiety diagnosis and was trying to cope with it, but other than that, I was enjoying a great life; I found the love of my life, and overall, I was happy. By the time I had my daughter, most of all those expectations had gone down the drain. After nine years in Atlanta, the city that I first arrived in 2002, we had to move to Birmingham, Alabama. One of the hardest things about that was leaving my friends behind; they were my only support system at that moment when I just had become a mom. My family and friends were far away and Eva was just three months old. While my husband was working, I was at home with my baby. I became a SAHM by choice. However, even while I was happy with my decision, there was a voice inside me that was telling me I wanted something more than just being with my daughter at home all day.

At the time, I started watching many of my friends advance in their careers and began to question my decision. I kept thinking about what could have happened if I had pursued my journalistic career instead. "What if I made the wrong choice?" I thought. I was unaware that little by little, I was separating myself from my real purpose. I fell in depression. I felt lonely, overwhelmed, exhausted, and insecure. It was overwhelming comparing myself with others, so I turned to the only thing I was sure I was good at: writing.

I decided to start a blog and get a book I had written published. Since I was a little girl, I have dreamt of writing books, but the dream got dormant for a while, and when the moment felt right, I said to myself "there is no better time than the present." So, while my daughter would take her naps and eventually went a few hours to daycare, I started my new personal path without even knowing it. I was posting in my blog periodically, and I was trying to get my book published, both things giving me a little of my life purpose back. I was also content with the way I was raising my daughter. Except for the times that anxiety and depression hit me, sometimes making me lose my patience, screaming at my little sweet baby cheeks who was learning to live in this chaotic world. Loneliness and isolation can produce reactions in you that you can't even imagine you could have. Her little eyes filled with love always brought me back to sanity. And I hugged her and remembered we needed each other. She gave me the strength to keep going in times when I thought I was going to lose my mind. I even started having ridiculous fights with relatives and friends. Now I know it was my anxiety monster reacting to those negative emotions I was incapable of correcting. My little achievements with my writings and watching my daughter grow in front of my eyes pulled me back together. But the anxiety monster was there, lurking and waiting for times to attack.

Meanwhile, I was discovering the publishing business, a world that is as tough as it gets. I had to learn many lessons from it, starting with dealing with rejection and judgment in ways I never imagined. My career was going nowhere, but I didn't care. I was following my voice, and writing was the only thing that kept me floating. The birth of my youngest changed everything, including my body, which ballooned an additional 62 pounds making me hate the person in the mirror. I managed to lose half of that weight, but my body, of course, would never be the same. Dealing with my self-esteem was extremely hard, and so my anxiety episodes began to be more frequent. Shortly after Erik was born, we moved back to Atlanta. I thought things were going to get better as I was going back to my support system, to my friends, and possibly to re-ignite my career. I was considering abandoning my writer's dreams; I was exhausted, so it seemed unattainable. I was happy to be back and oblivious to the fact that I was embarking on one of the hardest years of my life.

Here's how it goes. You have your first child, and it takes time until you can finally say, "I got this covered." You have your schedules set, and you start to gain some of your pre-motherhood life back, you start sleeping better and have already figured out what every single cry of your baby meant and how to handle her tantrums. "I am winning at motherhood," you finally think. "Hold my beer," says the universe, sending you baby #2 to completely change this. Not only your pregnancies are different, but the methods you use with number 1 most likely won't work with number 2 because they are entirely different human beings. Also, your relationship with your partner, if you have one, suffers a tremendous shift. You have to divide your focus into three people (plus the dog, in my case,) all while trying to make the most recent addition to the family survive.

Meanwhile, your new little one is still adjusting to the new family dynamic. You have less patience, and feel guilty because you are not giving your firstborn the attention you used to, and she is feeling it too. You have higher expectations for her behavior, sometimes forgetting she is just a toddler and not a second mom to your newborn baby. But oh, how proudly you say to your friends how she helps you change diapers and what a great big sister she is. Meanwhile, you forget what day of the week it is and good luck finding your keys or cellphone sometimes. Everyone keeps telling you how you can't forget about your partner, but you have no energy or are never in the mood for sex. All of this, while the anxiety monster is laughing in the corner, taunting you to lose your mind.

By the end of Erik's first year, I thought my family was falling apart. It was like that perfect storm and I didn't see how could I save myself because I believed I was losing myself to motherhood.

Alas, nothing could get any worse. Then hubby said once again, "we are moving." "Jacksonville, Florida," he muttered.

On the summer of 2014, we sent Eva to spend time with relatives and hubby, Erik and me went to check out Jacksonville. We spent two days in the city, but it only took us a few hours to know that moving was the right choice for us. Life has unexpected ways of fixing things around, and I was no longer scared of big changes. We packed again and moved from our big house to a much smaller apartment with a beautiful view of a marina. We initially thought that the place would be a temporary thing, but five years later, we are still there. Of course, we miss being in a big house, and maybe we will eventually... (I don't even want to say it or jinx it and now I don't like to make plans so the universe can keep surprising us!) Bottom line, the move helped us to be closer as a family and learn to use fewer things. We found that trips and experiences with our kids gave us more quality time than a large basement or big backyard. Plus, the beach is so close, it's always a blessing to go even if it is for a short walk. Once we moved, our daughter started the "big kids" school, and things began to fall into place, like a Tetris game. The thing about big storms is that they always end. They are necessary. They can move you and make you sick, and you end up trying to protect yourself from the lighting and carefully avoiding the perils and dangers of the violent breeze and giant waves. No storm is eternal, though. Even when they destroy things around, they also nourish you and clean your air. Just what had happened to me after that chaotic year in Atlanta.

Once accommodated and acclimated in Jacksonville, I resumed my dreams, but this time around I was determined to do something different. I was first going to commit to fixing the relationship with one person only: Me. I needed to fulfill my dreams and needs, and take matters in my own hands.

I decided I was not going to be labeled anymore. Paola is just one person, who happens to be a mom, a writer, a wife, a daughter, a sister, a friend, and so many other things. When we moved, I started a path of reinventing myself with anxiety and everything on board. I started loving myself, even in my darkest days, with all my imperfections, in any circumstances, in every mood. It took me a while to realize I was where I was supposed to be every single time to become who I needed to be. Every choice I made, every challenge, every battle, and every triumph had and kept having a reason. A lot of things happened once I took that decision to commit to myself, and one of those things was having the courage to self-publishing my first book.

The day the prints arrived at my home was one of the happiest of my life. A materialized dream gives you satisfaction beyond comprehension. But there was something even better than that, and I will not forget the look in my children's eyes the day I presented my book at the International Book Fair of Bogota (FILBO), one of the most important book fairs in Latin America. When you fulfill a dream, you are setting an example for your kids that no one else can give them. You are showing them what life is all about, and those are lessons they will never forget, no matter how little they are. These lessons fuel them from a very early age to fulfill their own dreams while feeding you to keep dreaming and fighting for even more ideas. What makes you happy and shine should be your goal for you and your family too.

Writing and publishing that book was one of the hardest things I have ever done. But it marked my path. I showed myself that I could accomplish whatever I set out to do. Now I have six books (including this one!) and keep on writing. I started my healing process from anxiety and now I can keep the monster at bay. When I transformed into my better version and realized that is progress and not perfection, what makes a person happy, I felt like a better mother and partner to my husband. By all means, I am not saying my life is 100% figured out. I still have challenges and goals, new dreams to conquer, and remember, I still have that little monster around. But life throws experiences so you can learn the lessons.

I also think that I am lucky I have a partner that has been growing with me since the day we met. My husband and I have been through thick and thin and have endured many things together, including my anxiety battles. Understanding that a relationship is never perfect was also crucial in my path of self-discovery. Knowing that you decide to co-create a life with someone that is different but that somehow shares similar objectives, and that is not our responsibility to make each other happy but share our own happiness with one another. When you understand that you have to be a team where no one is above but everyone has to have roles, your family starts swimming in a wonderful pool of surprises. You have good years and bad years but your decision to love that person and to see him in that light can make a big difference in your relationship, no matter the challenges or the disagreements between you. And that is how I am choosing from now on to see everyone and everything around me, through the light and love I can feel for them. Loving is more than a feeling but a choice, and you can take it.

Another thing to remember is the self-care factor. During the quarantine in 2020, it was like a mandatory statement everywhere: you shall practice self-care. Here is the thing. Self-care is different for everybody. Some might feel is exercise, others to put makeup and get dressy, others just having a few minutes of solitude. If you find out what are your needs, and do what you have to do to make yourself happy and keep your anxiety monster at bay, be unapologetic about how you handle your self-care. Your priority is not making everyone else comfortable and happy, but fulfilling whatever it is that you need to take away some of the new anxieties and pressures that life brings. Maybe just by acknowledging this, we could see other mothers differently.

Do you remember Morpheus in *The Matrix*? Let's use him. Imagine him in front of you when you have to face a situation that causes you anxiety, a problem, a challenge, or when you have a dream that you want to make real... You can take the blue pill. Concentrate on the fear it produces you, making the situation overwhelming and uncontrollable, fixating on the outcome, making you believe that a solution or a dream come true is impossible. Or you can take the red pill, choosing to see the opportunity as your path to self-discovering, focusing on the feelings, knowing there is guidance inside you fueled by love and compassion, that is not only heeling you but also providing you with the inspiration and the strength to take action and fight for what you want. Yes, you may have to fight like Neo, but "what if I told you" that choosing this pill can also give you his ability to dodge bullets? The choice is yours.

 LESSON: Prioritize the relationship you have with yourself and never forget about your dreams. Notice how important you are, knowing that even in the darkest moments, you can be the light if you choose to see life through love instead of fear.

TIPS:

- Make a list of your top dreams. Then put three actions you can take right now to make them come true.
- Make also a list of the feelings that attaining that dream can awake in you. Let yourself feel those as if you were already having your wish fulfilled.
- Use visualization. See yourself already having those dreams fulfilled and notice the change of energy and emotions once you see yourself attaining such goals. Now, believe that this is possible because it is!
- Self-care is different for everyone. It can be exercise, writing, putting makeup on, even as simple as taking a shower, dedicate a few minutes a day to your self-care.
- **The more love you give to yourself, the more love you'll have to share with your family. LOVE YOURSELF, FIRST.** Write a vivid description of yourself. If you are not there, then a positive description of who you want to become as if you are already there. Read it daily in the morning and night or whenever you feel down. Remember, you are the blood.

EDUCATE YOURSELF AND OTHERS ABOUT ANXIETY AS MUCH AS YOU CAN

"Always pass on what you have learned."
–Yoda, Star Wars

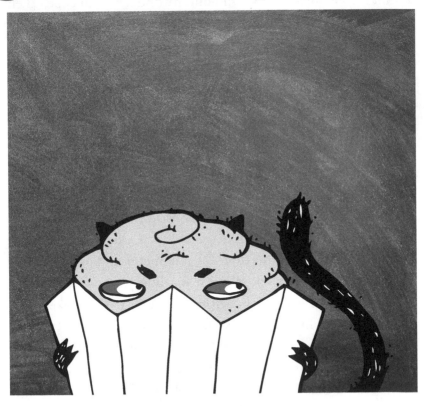

There was a moment that I can't forget. It was a few years ago before I became so public with my anxiety condition. I came back home from dropping the kids at school after one of my worst panic attacks. I had no strength, neither physically, mentally, or emotionally. I was drained; I was tired of this monster and I just started to cry. Lying on the floor filled with pain and agony, I began to cry, "Why me?" I didn't understand why I had to suffer from anxiety, or why I couldn't find a way to cope. Then I was filled with anger. I start yelling at God. I was asking him to stop. I was telling him I refused to have this test. I was there in the darkness, trying to find the light, and I realized then that the reason I couldn't see it was because I was looking for it in the wrong place. We can't see the light while searching it outside. We need to ignite the fire inside of us first to create it and be guided by it.

You can call it instinct, inspiration, or maybe it was "the force." I decided to write about it, so I sat down, and out of me came my first post, The Truth of the Anxious Mom. I didn't even doubt about posting it on my blog. I knew it was extremely personal, and that I was opening the door for judgments and opinions, but I didn't care. I needed to do it and it was liberating. When I wrote it a lot of things happened. Before I posted it, I felt like I was the only person in the world suffering from this. Then I started receiving messages from people I didn't know, and others that I did, telling me that they were amazed and moved by my words because it was exactly how they were feeling. A lot of these messages weren't public, though. People chose to write to me directly, and I understood them and respected their decision. I realized that the problem is that we are so afraid to speak and tell others what is happening. We think we are alone, and just the fact of knowing that someone else is also having a similar experience gives you hope. You start realizing it happens to others, and you can feel empathy. We are never alone. But compassion is not enough. If we don't help each other, there is no point. We can't just vent and sink together. We need to lift each other. Something occurred to me: maybe telling our stories of anxiety can help people to feel more included and show them that they are not alone. Perhaps those same stories can help those who know someone with anxiety to get closer and understand how that person feels and will provide them with tools to become more compassionate toward people that suffer from this or any other mental illness. Maybe these stories will show others that they don't have to hide, that we can heal, and that it is possible to cope with this condition.

That was the beginning of all of this. That was the beginning of Momxious and a new purpose as a writer, a mission that was overcast at first, but now is crystal clear, and I can't doubt or deny it.

I strongly believe that each of us has a purpose here. Also, that we are so connected to each other that somehow all our intentions are intertwined. If you are reading this book is because you were meant to read it. I don't know if you suffer from anxiety or know someone who does, but there's a reason you now have this information, and now you can help my purpose. Create awareness about this condition and provide tools that can be helpful for others to cope with it. It's that simple. I am not sure which of the methods I have used can be helpful to you or someone you know, because anxiety is different for everyone. However, just by not remaining silent, we are not only educating others about this condition but we are also helping to end the stigma around mothers and mental health. By letting others know they are not alone, we are helping. By being compassionate to another mom struggling, we are helping.

The work of a creator serves a personal purpose first. When I wrote this book I was moved to find my own declarations and finally screaming to the universe my commitment to feeling good. It was an exhilarating process, I was healing through it, it was cathartic and liberating. Then I was inspired to releasing my words to the world and they might have a purpose beyond, I can't be sure. They might speak to you or not and your interpretation of them is only yours. If it does, I hope you take the rules of this manifesto and make use of them to change your life and the life of others around you. My wish is that my words inspire you and give you hope and comfort. We are just getting started and there is much more that we can do together.

Mothers already suffer from isolation. We know that we wouldn't change our role from any other. Being a mom has given me more meaning than I could ever imagine, but it's a hard job. So, I propose something. Let's be partners in this. Let's support each other and hold each other's hands, respecting other mom's choices along the way, even if we don't agree, or if we do things differently. We are raising future generations, so it's in our hands to provide them a world were compassion is flowing. Each of us has a different way to raise our kids, and that's okay. We don't have to fight about it but understand that we are doing the best. We need to stop searching for perfection and start aiming for progress.

I also strongly encourage you to talk about your anxiety. You don't need to be a writer or have a blog. You don't need to be as public as I was. You can decide how you want to talk about this. Many groups in social media offer support for moms with anxiety if what you are looking for is a place to express your emotions or blow off some steam. Or you can join mine, Momxious, support for the anxious mom on Facebook. It's a safe space where you can talk and find encouragement. You can also talk to your family, even to your kids, and help them understand. If you have the possibility or the ability to speak to larger groups about this, please do. You never know who is out there trying to figure this out, trying to understand why they feel like this and what they can do to feel better. You need to know also that there are several organizations and programs out there for moms like us.

Another thing I recommend is having a friend on-call, the Anxiety Distractor Buddy. I mentioned this in a previous chapter and I want to explain to you more about it. You don't even have to have a panic attack to call that person. I see it this way. A few years ago, before motherhood, my husband encouraged me to learn how to dive. Despite all odds, I finished my training, and I even got the advanced diver certification. One of the rules for diving is that you need to ALWAYS have a buddy with you. It's vital for safety, in case you have an emergency or there is something wrong with your equipment, your buddy is there to help you, or you to help them. Plus, it's always more fun when you dive with someone else. Anxiety can feel like drowning. Sometimes your tank runs out of oxygen, or you get lost or terrified, and your buddy can take you afloat. That person doesn't necessarily need to suffer from anxiety too. It can be anyone you trust. Anyone you can call in your darkest moments. Choose that person wisely and nurture your relationship with him or her. I told you already that it can also be your pet. My dog Khan, an 11-year-old Siberian husky has been there for me several times, always ready to listen, always giving me that comfort look than only a pet can give you. I have no doubt that the soul of a pet chooses you to bring you more than companionship but lessons of unconditional and pure love. When I have no one around Khan is the perfect ADB and will be the best as long as he lives.

The important thing you need to know is that there are ways that you can express yourself and not feel alone in this fight. You aren't. Talking helps. Plus, you and I know how difficult the system can be for therapy and treatments. I endured that myself. Searching for a therapist was like finding a job. And let's not even talk about the costs. Hopefully, by creating awareness, we will create some change.

We can stop the taboo and the perpetuation of the false perfection image of motherhood. We can end the stigma of talking about mental health. Trust me; you can contribute to the conversation and benefit your healing. You will discover a power that is undeniable in everyone, the power of co-create.

Most of the time, people fear what they don't know. To stop worrying about anxiety for yourself and others, you need to start educating yourself as much as you can. Fortunately for us, we now have the technology on our side and just one click away. Share important information with others. The more we know, the more we help. That's also a way to grow and heal.

 LESSON: You are not alone in this fight. Your voice can contribute to your own healing as well as the others around you. The more you know the monster, the higher the chance you will be able to defeat it, but we can't do this alone. We need each other.

 TIPS:
- Join a support group on social media.
- Spread awareness in any way you can.
- Talk to your loved ones, as it will help you to recognize your triggers, making it easier to be prepared and proactive about your healing.

MAKE YOUR ANXIETY MONSTER A LIFE MASTER

 "Always two there are, no more, no less. A master and an apprentice."

—Yoda, Star Wars

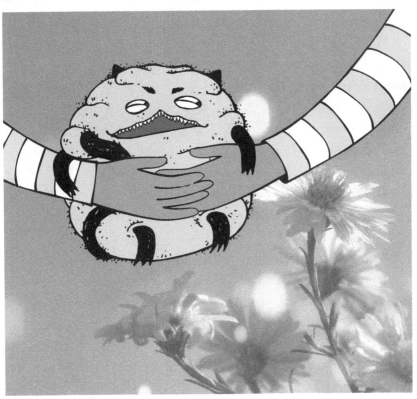

By now, you should recognize there is a monster. Having a visual image of the beast can help you change your relationship with anxiety. This personification can also encourage you to stop fearing the monster. You can choose to nurture it or not. Remember, it feeds from your fears (like Pennywise!) The more you feed it, the more it grows and it becomes stronger. So, how about you decide to love the monster and let its presence be an opportunity for learning and growing? It's not impossible, and here's why.

When you hate something or someone, you are just filling yourself with a tremendous amount of negative energy. The monster feels your hate and uses it to cling to you, like a leech. If you acknowledge its presence but choose to heal through love instead of fear and hate, it will lose its power because the energy that surrounds you has shifted. That positive energy has healing power and can attract other positive things into your life. When you choose to take action from a place of love, you will get inspired to find solutions. When you do it from a position of fear or anger, you won't see results.

For example, remember how many times you have recovered from a panic attack. You know for a fact that it takes a tremendous amount of strength to recover from one of those. You might not recognize it at the moment, but it was you and only you who created that strength. You have two choices. Hate the panic attack and wait until it appears again, fearing and expecting, disregarding your victory or, choose to love the strength that you created and that had made you recover time after time. Acknowledge, with conviction, that you can be strong as often as it takes, and that you can birth strength in other situations. Are you not convinced? If you decide to face a fear, like me in the roller coaster, next time you have to face a similar situation, you will kill the monster's need to feed on your fear because it's not there anymore. Love the strength, but love the monster too because it was somehow through it that you realized that strength in you.

Love the lessons learned in every battle. Love the rejections, the obstacles, the doors that were closed to you, because they were closing the wrong path for you, allowing yourself to find the right one. If you cloud your soul with defeat and hate, you won't see that path. However, we need those losses, the darkness, the bad days, to appreciate what matters, the light inside of us. Remember how in *Inside Out*, Joy was desperately trying to save Sadness? If you haven't seen it, grab popcorn and do it, is a fun movie to see with your kids, and also explains a lot about emotions and empathy. The point is that we all experience duality, but we can choose which of the two sides will be more significant at the end of the day.

Anxiety can teach you many things about yourself. By battling the monster, you can acquire many tools, like in a game with many levels. In the beginning, you just have one or two weapons to defend yourself, but then on level 12, you are going to have more skills than Liam Neeson in the movie *Taken* and so on. Even if the monster never disappears, what matters is that you know exactly what to do when it shows up.

The reason why I created this monster was to allow myself to exteriorized it. Personification can be helpful because we can relate to something we see more quickly than if it is invisible. We all have to deal with monsters. We can choose to fight them; however, monsters like anxiety are difficult to defeat, but not impossible. The first step is deciding to stop fearing the beast and look at it with different eyes. It came into your life with a purpose like other things that surround you. It can be a life master if you allow the lessons that anxiety gives you to work in your favor. When you turn your monster into a master, soon you will be the master of your life. Here is a lesson behind every time you feel anxious. You have this condition but you have the strength to overcome it. Never doubt your capacities and don't let anyone make you doubt in yourself.

Now that you have a visual, you can give it a name. Own it, not the other way around. Go ahead! Claim it and make it work for you. I know it isn't easy. I know it will take time. But you can do it. You can come to any chapter of this book and any declaration anytime you want. I also keep posting fun memes, information, new tools, methods, and all sort of motivational content in my social media channels, newsletter, and Momxious Community. I promise I am here with you. I will not abandon you. I will continue fighting this fight along with you, developing more books, products, community, and awareness. Stay tuned and follow me for more things to come! Before you go I will leave you with a prayer. (If you don't want to call it prayer, call it a poem, inspirational quote, words on a paragraph, whatever you prefer.) You can say this whenever you feel anxious or whenever you need strength.

I am a being of light. I carry inside a strength that nothing and no one can take away from me.

As my path goes by, I am taking the lessons of each day, knowing they were necessary for my learning and growth.

I am not alone, and I remember we all need each other and that all our purposes are interconnected.

I am the best I can be, and that is the only value where I need to put my focus on.

I refuse to see anxiety as my enemy. I recognize it as a master that is providing me tools and lessons to be the person I came here to be. For my children, for my family, for myself, for those around me.

I am love, and through love, I heal.

ABOUT THE AUTHOR

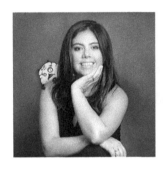

Paola B. Sur is an award-winning author, originally from Colombia. Mother of two, blogger, and mostly a dreamer. She loves fiction fantasy, coffee, and soccer. Her experiences as a mom living with anxiety started the blog series named *Momxious*, which later developed into *The Anxious Mom Manifesto*, attracting hundreds of followers into her social media accounts who felt Paola's experiences incredibly relatable. Her first novel El Lago de los Milagros (2016) (Spanish version) is an Award Winning Book at the International Latino Book Awards 2017, a finalist in the categories of Best Fantasy Novel, and Best First Book/Children and Youth.

The Lake of Miracles (2017) obtained second place at the Latino Books into Movie Awards, finalist in the Fantasy Category.

Paola recently published Shorty Tales (Cuentitos) a collection of short bilingual stories intended to promote multi-language learning through storytelling experiences. Also, she published her most recent fantasy novel Un Mundo Increíble (Spanish Version)

Her work has appeared on *Ser Padres, Mundo Hispánico, Scary Mommy, and First Coast Magazine,* and she was Editor-in-Chief of *Muévelo Magazine.* She earned a Master of Arts in Communication from Georgia State University in 2011.

Paola currently lives in Jacksonville, Florida with her husband and kids. You can follow her @paobsur and reach her at www.paolasur.com www.momxious.com

CPSIA information can be obtained
at www.ICGtesting.com
Printed in the USA
JSHW032136280421
14077JS00008B/278